I0472362

PSYCHIATRISTS ILLUSTRATED
CARTOONS SUMMARIZING THE
BEHAVIOR OF PSYCHIATRISTS

Kenneth Kramer

PSYCHIATRISTS ILLUSTRATED

Copyright © 2019 Kenneth Kramer
All rights reserved.
ISBN: 9781095482971

DEDICATION

To the men who shoulder the world's weight and to my spirited wife who lifts more than most of them.

CONTENTS

ACKNOWLEDGMENTS

To world class artists, Horst Dubiel, Jonathan Brown, Rick Rogers and Verde! Your brilliant creations are much appreciated. I can't wait to see what you come up with for the 2nd edition of this book!

To my mother, who taught me to stand up to bullies. To my father, who whispered to me: "Quit show'n off and just bust the ball!"

And to my special and lovely wife, Trish, who listens to me, no matter how many times I repeat myself and is seemingly always interested though I don't see how on earth that is possible!

THE APA
AMERICAN PSYCHIATRIST ASSOCIATION

Psychs

by Kramer & Brown

"I started listening and stopped prescribing. They kicked me out!"

The "Shrink" Tank
by Verde

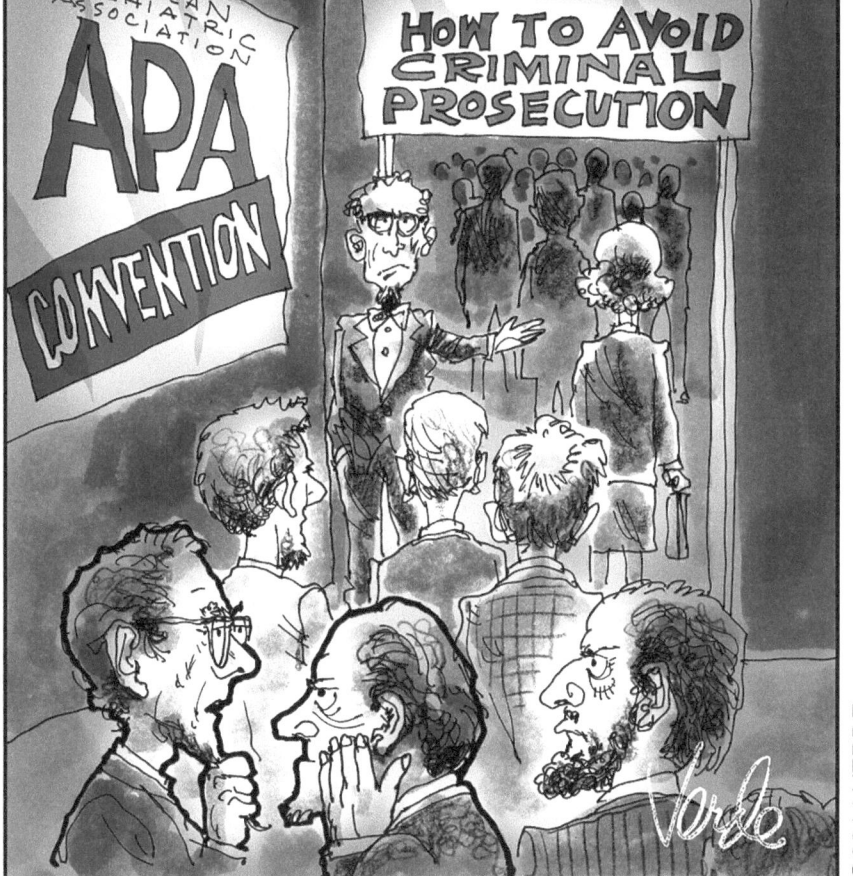

"I hope they cover sexual misconduct."

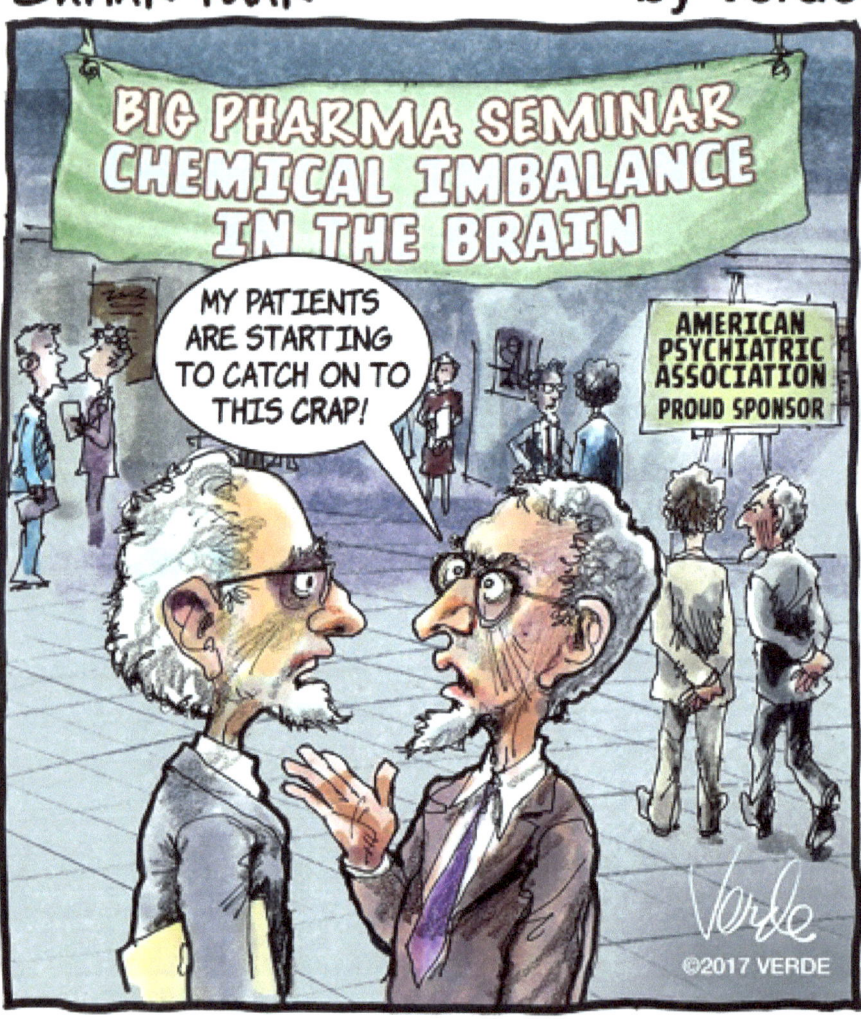

The "Shrink" Tank   by Verde

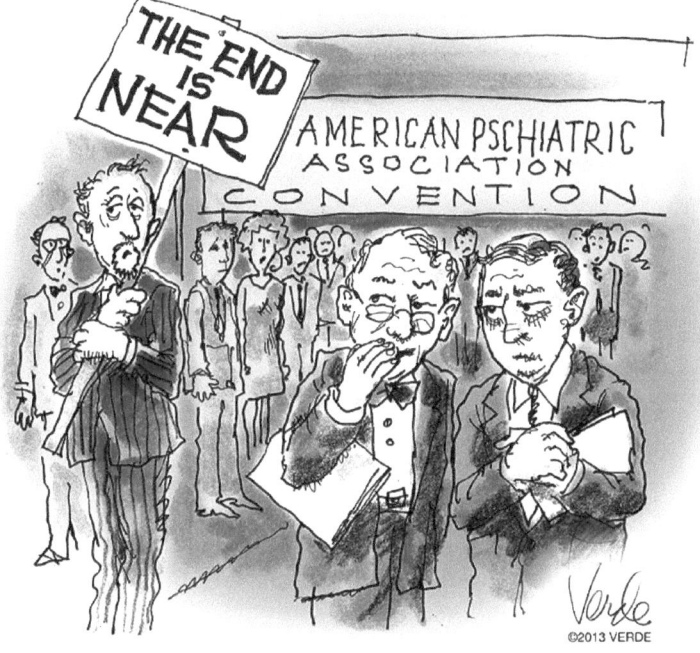

"Ever since the DSM was cancelled by NIMH ... the doctor's been acting odd.

COURTS

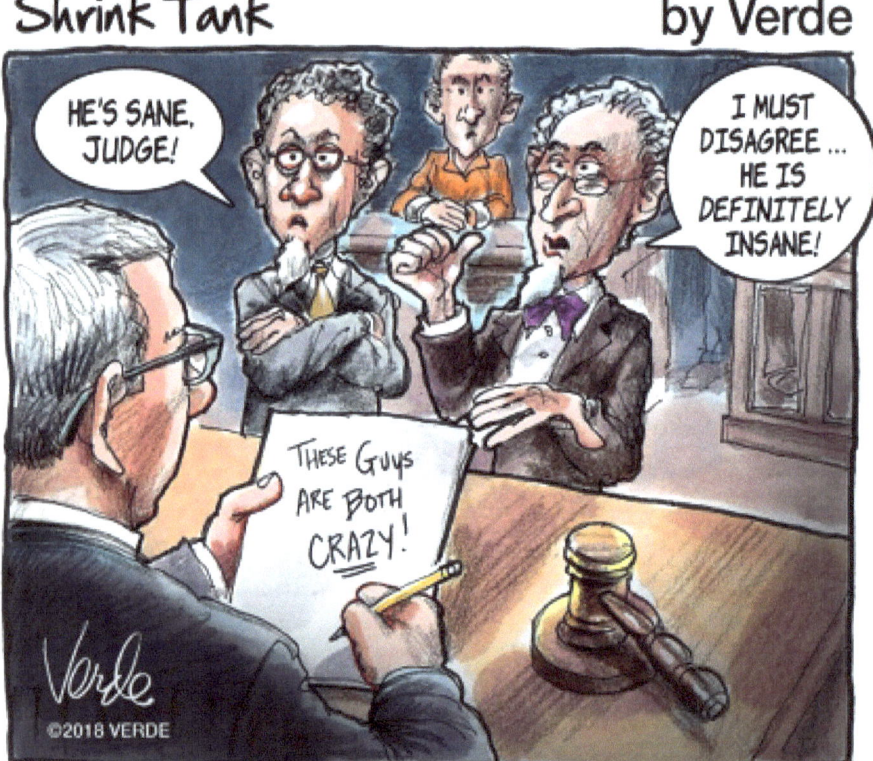

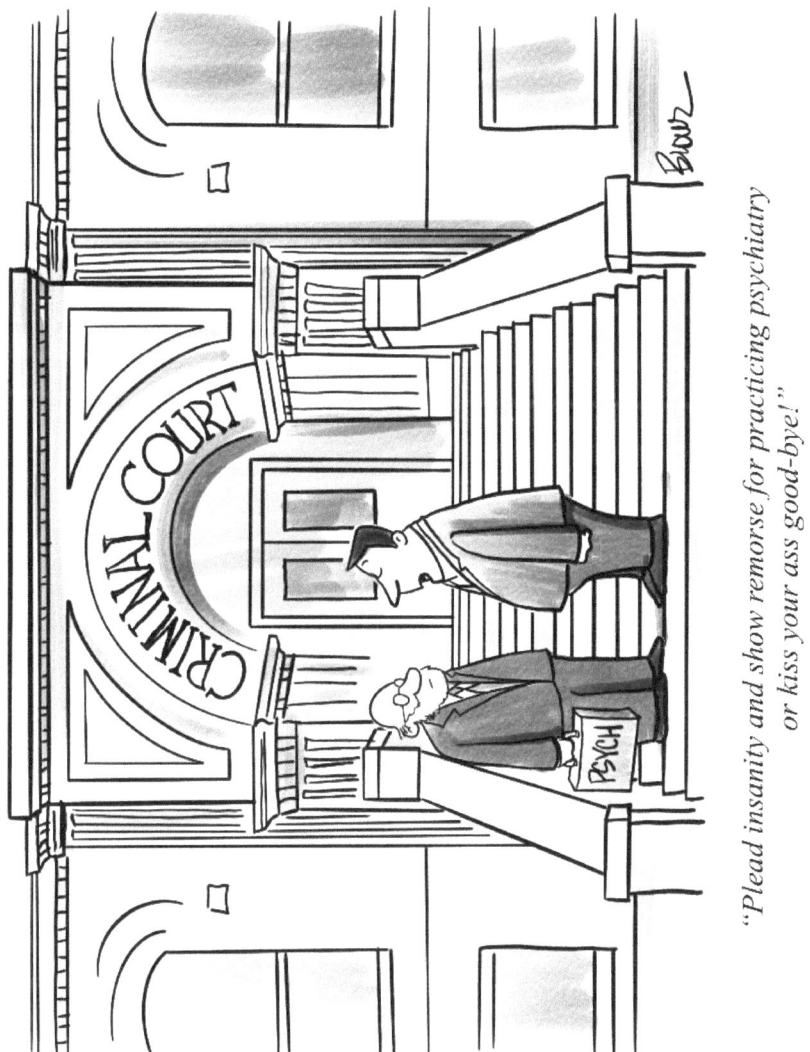

"Plead insanity and show remorse for practicing psychiatry or kiss your ass good-bye!"

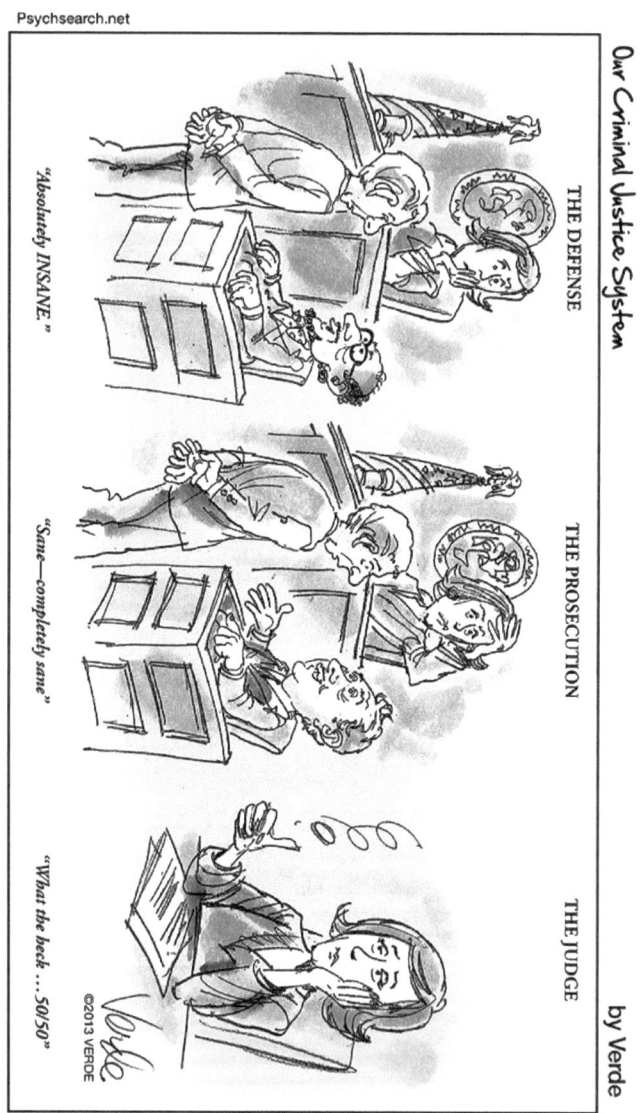

FUNDING

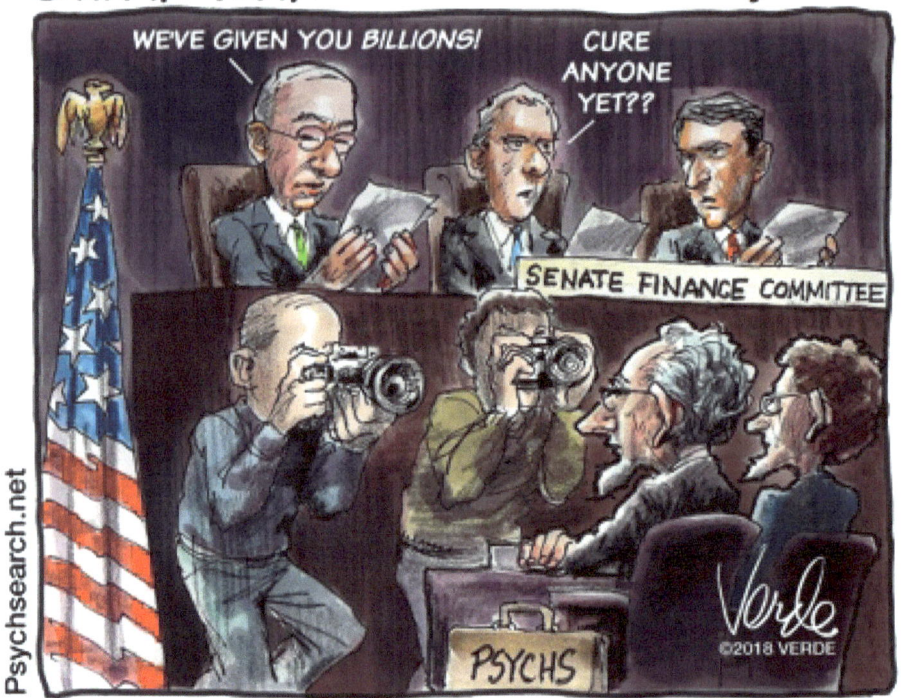

"No Senator … we need *more* funding."

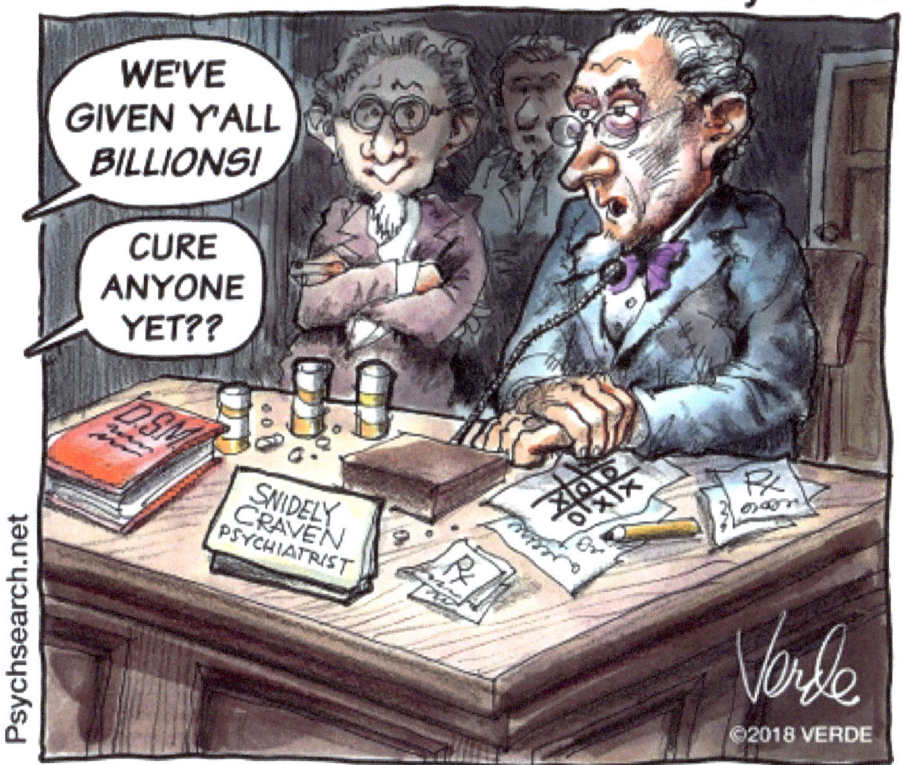

"No Senator … we need more funding."

DSM
DIAGNOSTIC & STATISTICAL MANUAL OF MENTAL DISORDERS
THE "BIBLE" OF PSYCHIATRISTS
[CONTAINS NO STATISTICS AND
HAS NO CURES]

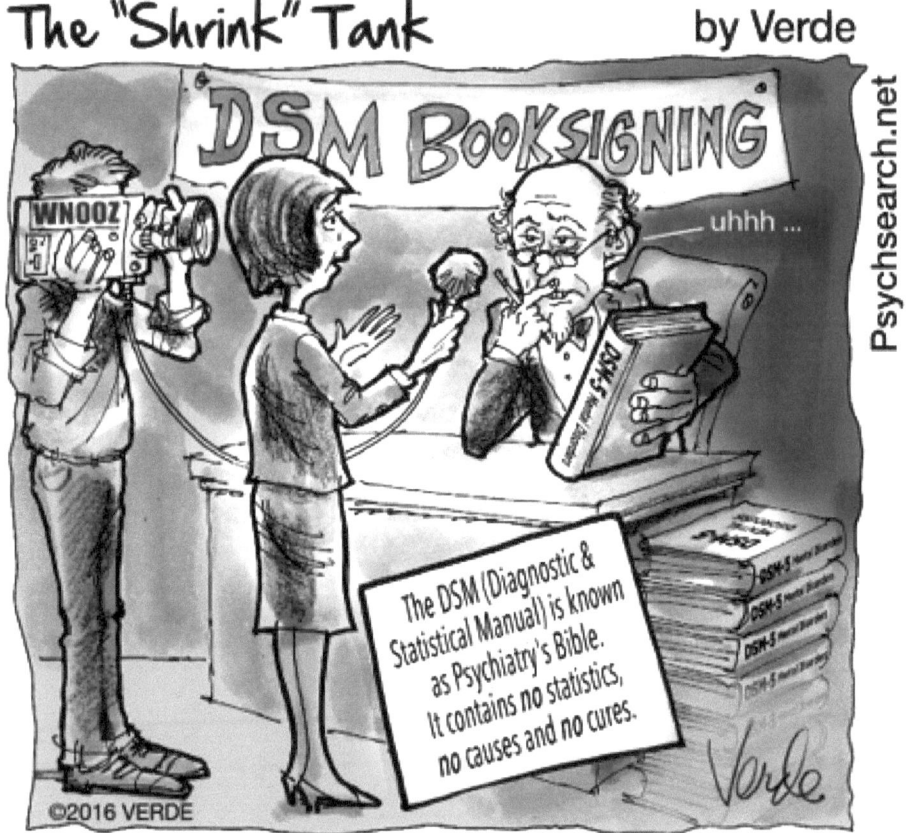

So Mr. Psychiatrist ... have you ever *cured* anyone?

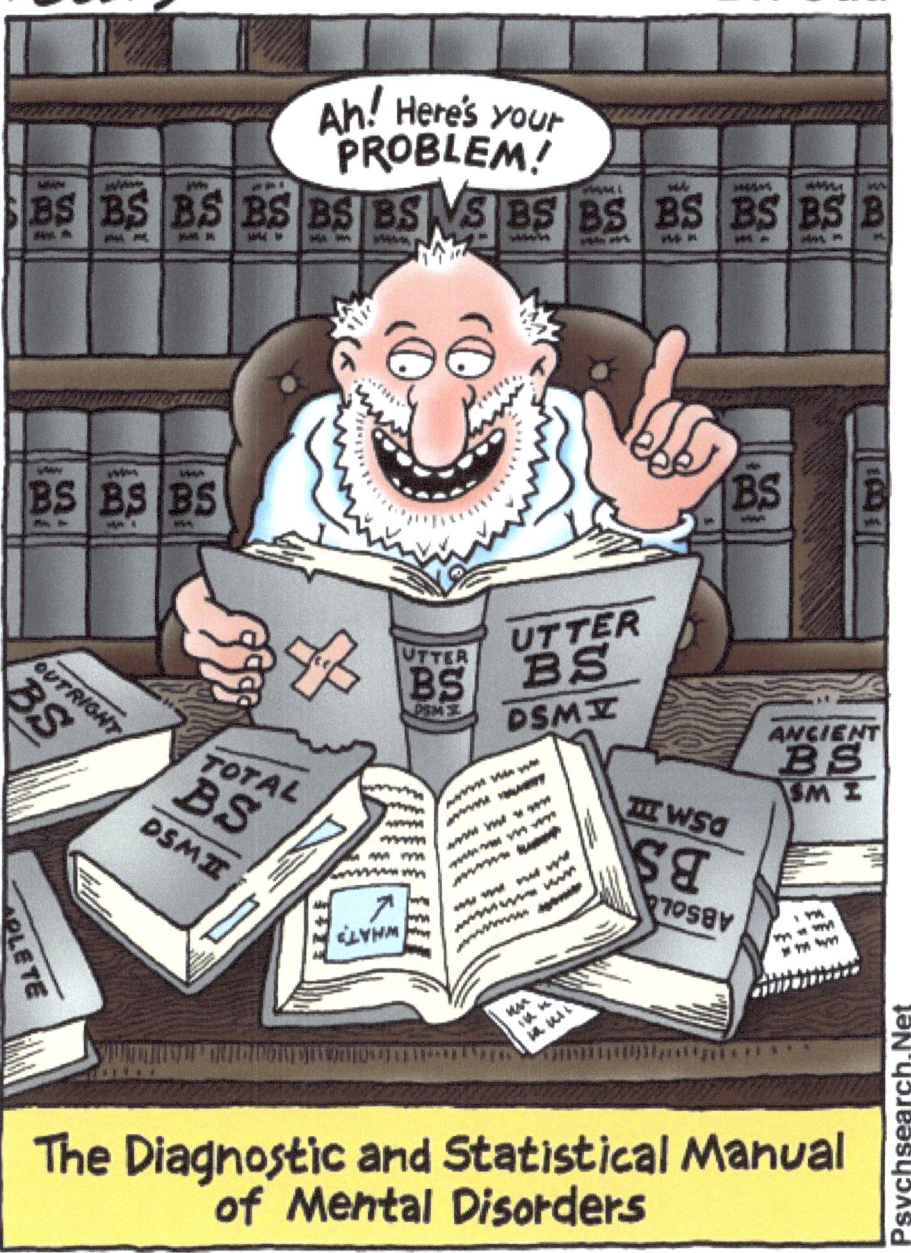

The Diagnostic and Statistical Manual
of Mental Disorders

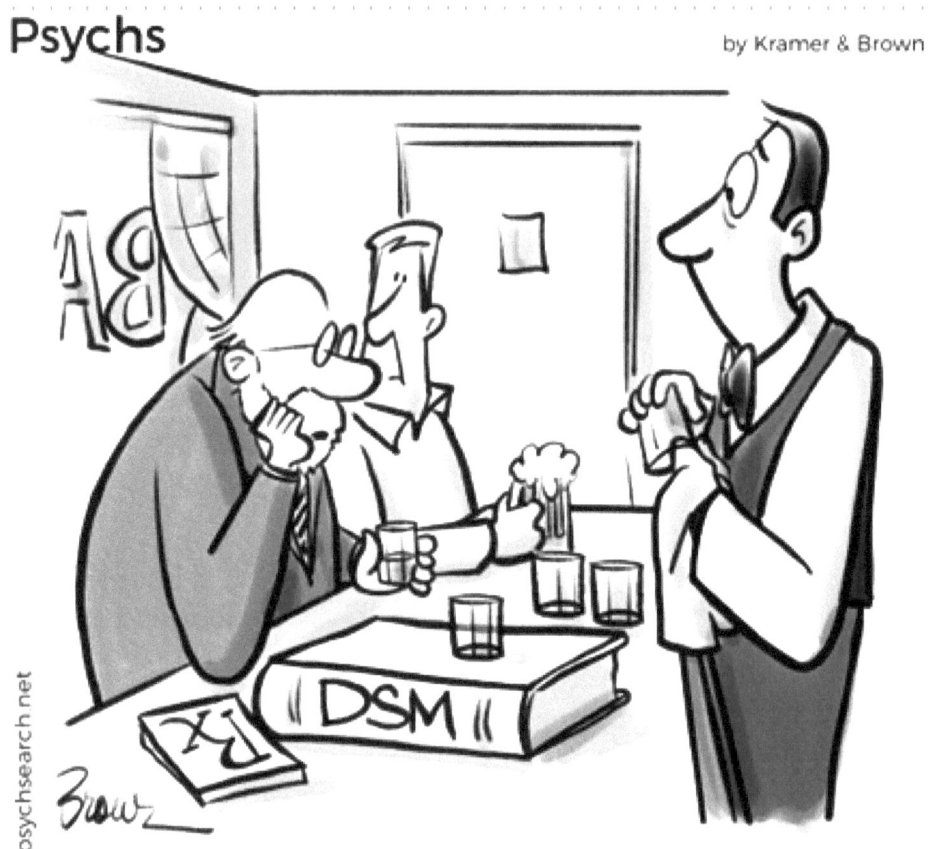

"Of course, you can't do anything about insanity, really, so it doesn't matter what I do, does it?"

Maybe spelling it out might help the appreciation?

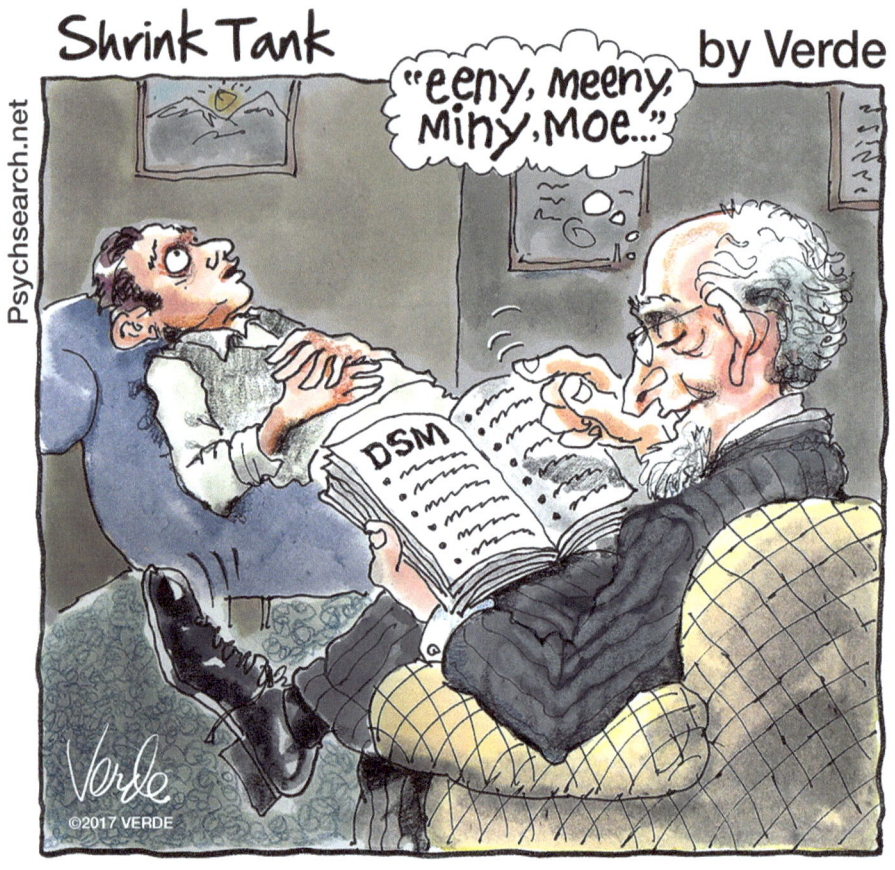

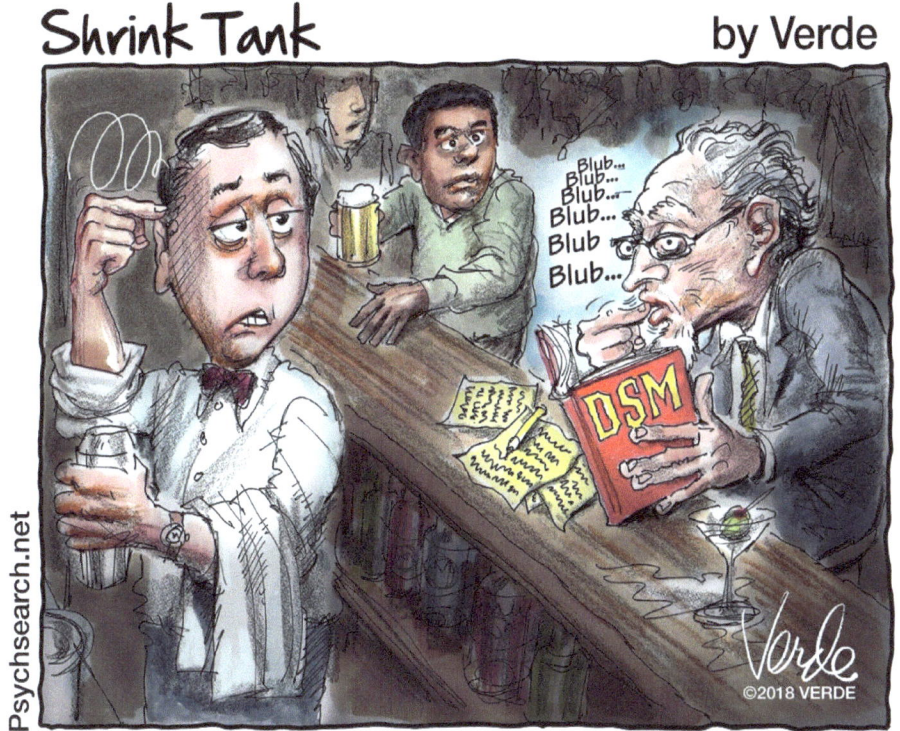

"Psychiatrists are THEEE nuttiest!"

ADHD

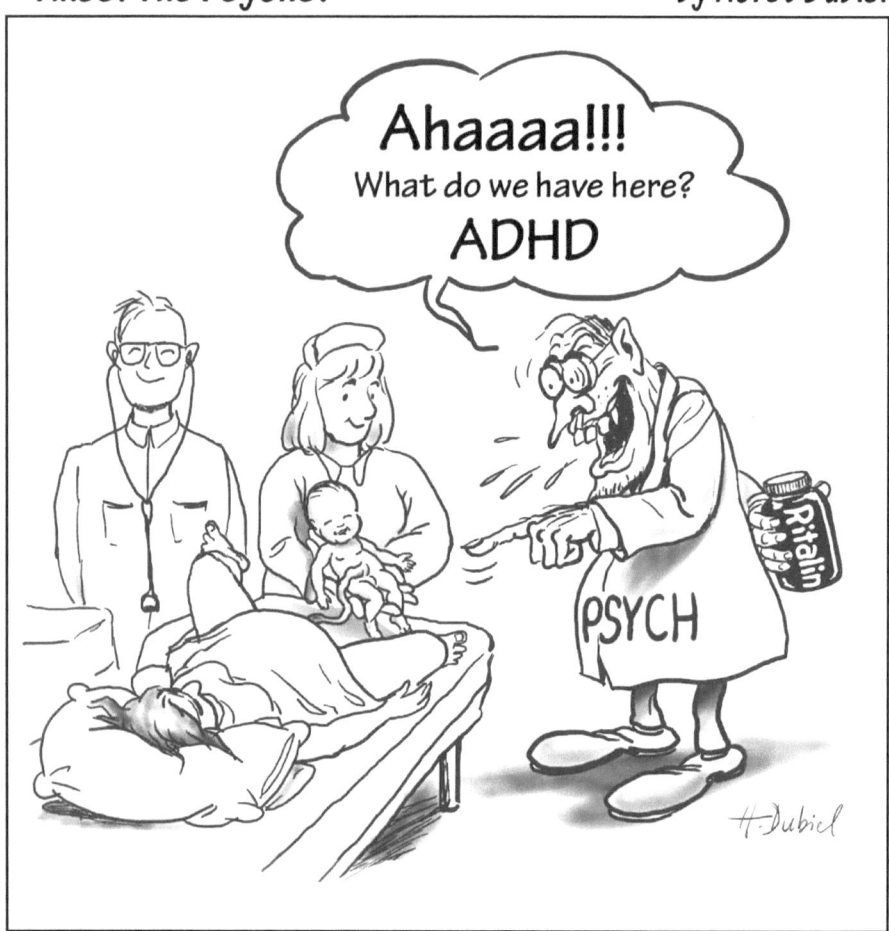

Psychs

by Kramer & Brown

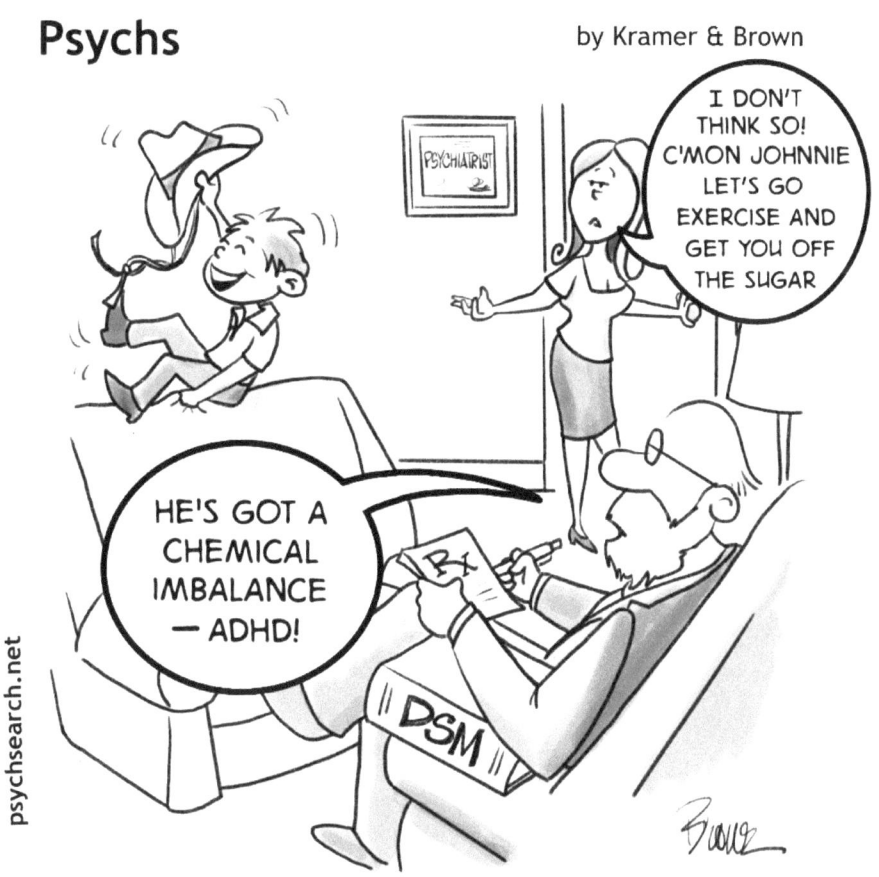

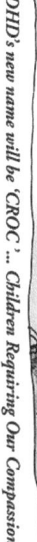

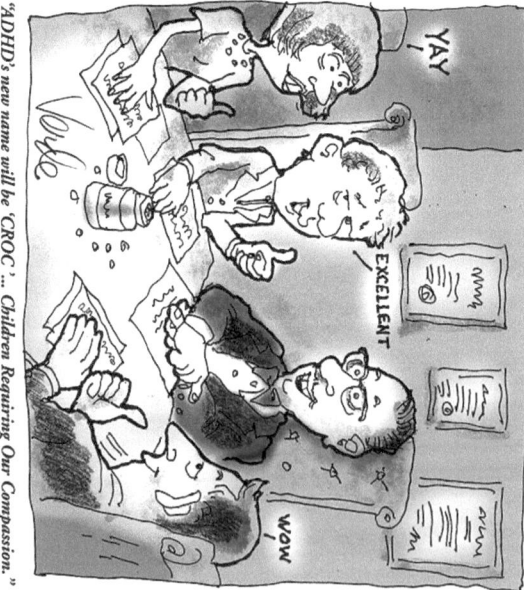

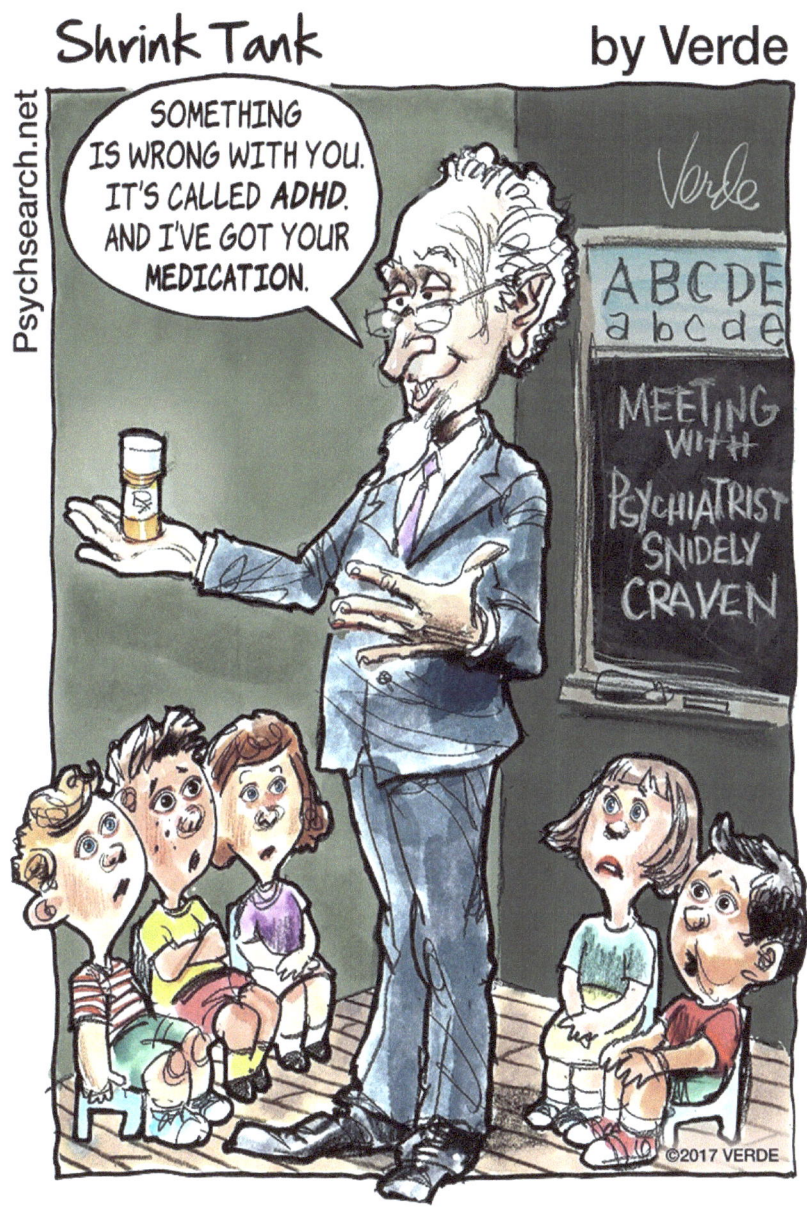

School Bully

BIG PHARMA

Psychs

by Kramer & Brown

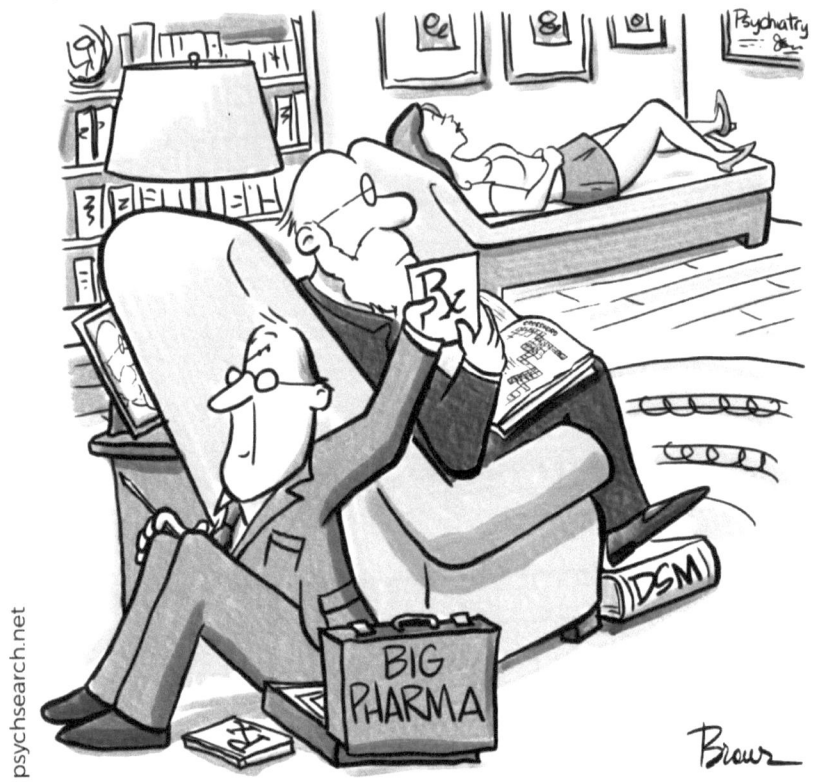

psychsearch.net

COLLUSION

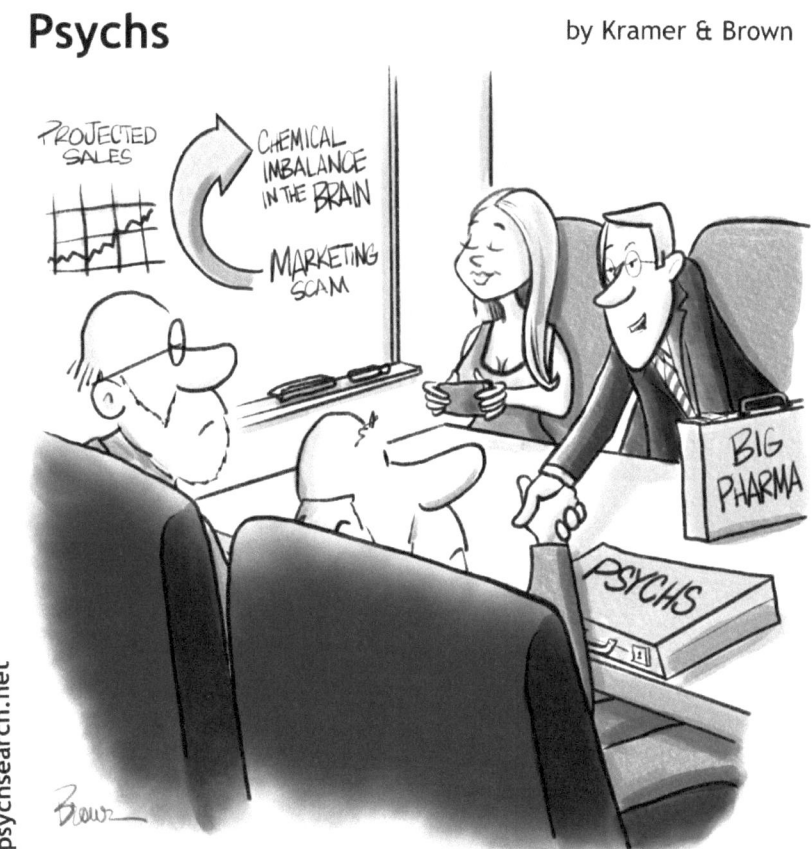

*"You dream up another bogus mental disorder.
We'll come up with the drugs."*

Psychs

by Kramer & Brown

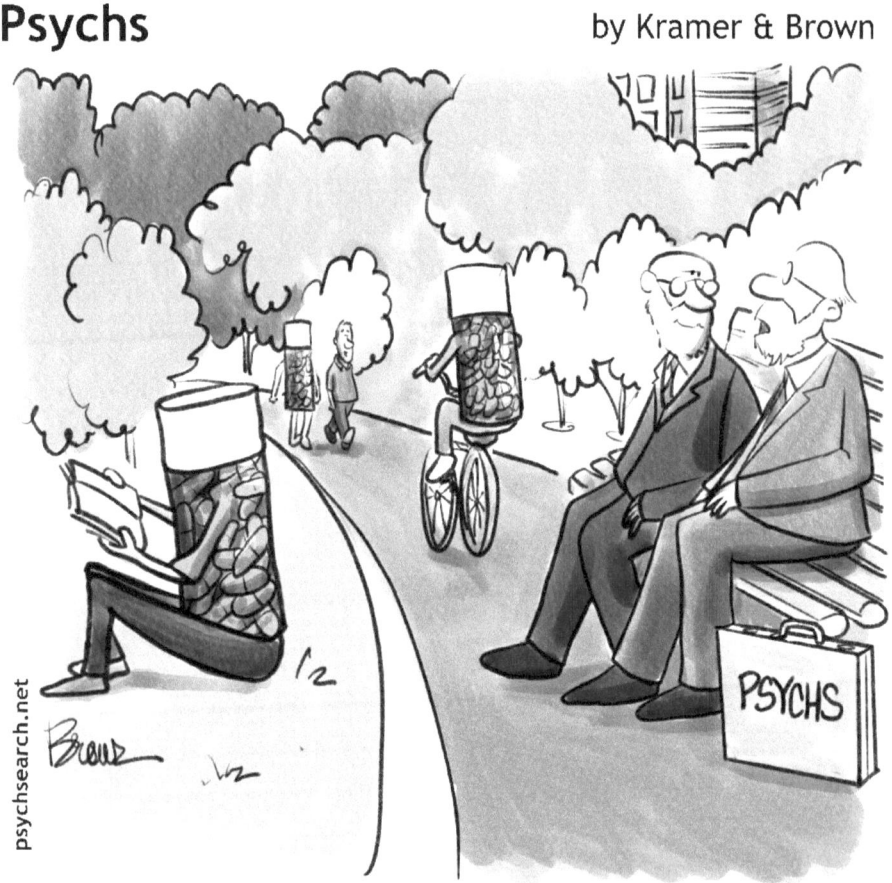

*Ya know, without Big Pharma's **Direct-to-Consumer Advertising**, we'd be extinct!"*

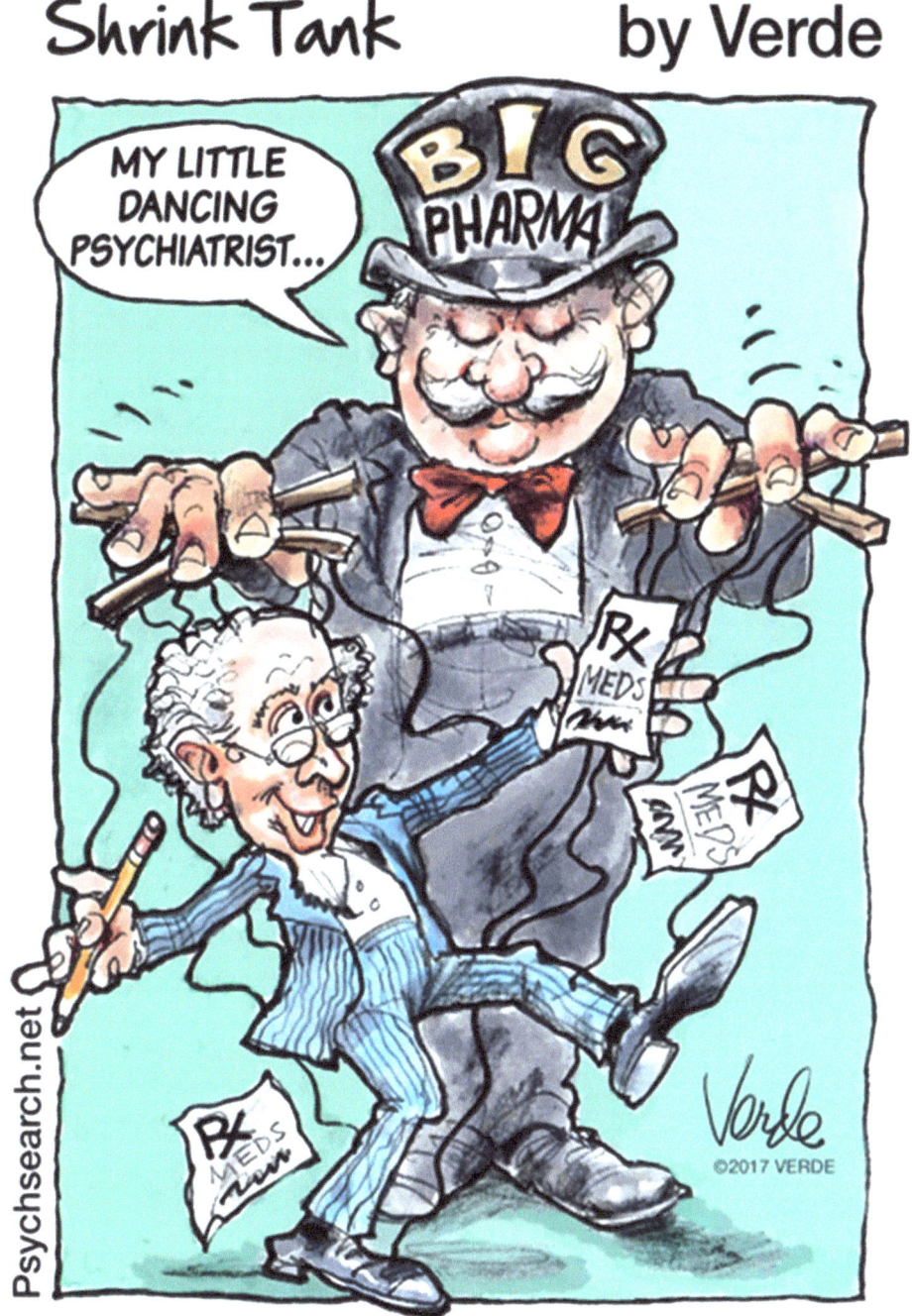

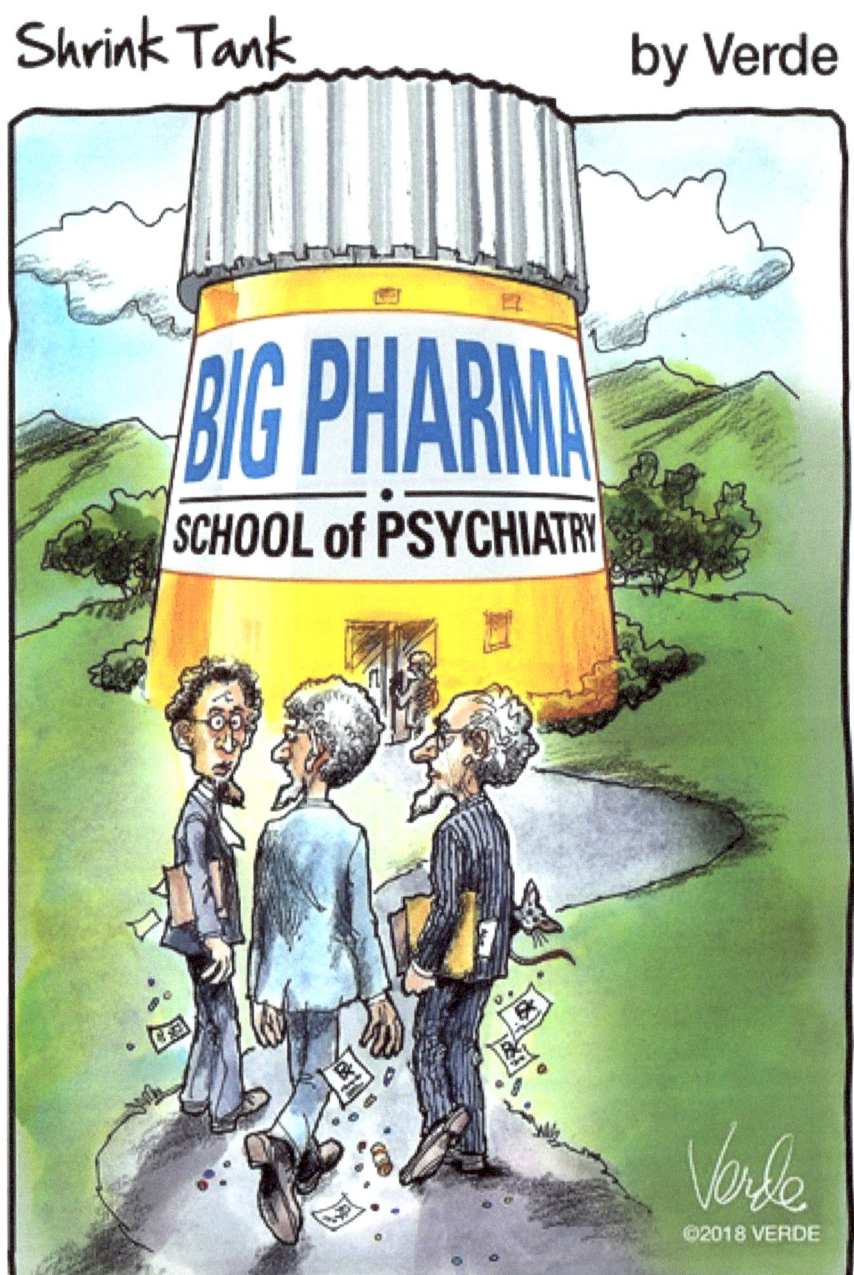

A marriage made in Hell

Shrink Tank

by Verde

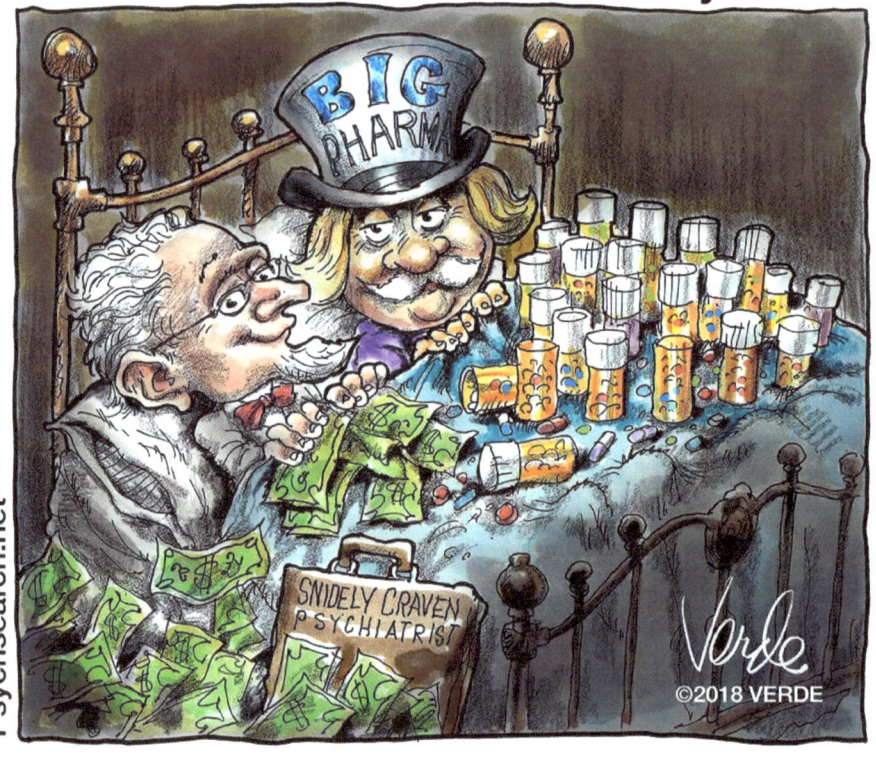

Bedfellows

SHOCK TREATMENT
ELECTROCONVULSIVE 'THERAPY"
ECT

The "Shrink" Tank by Verde

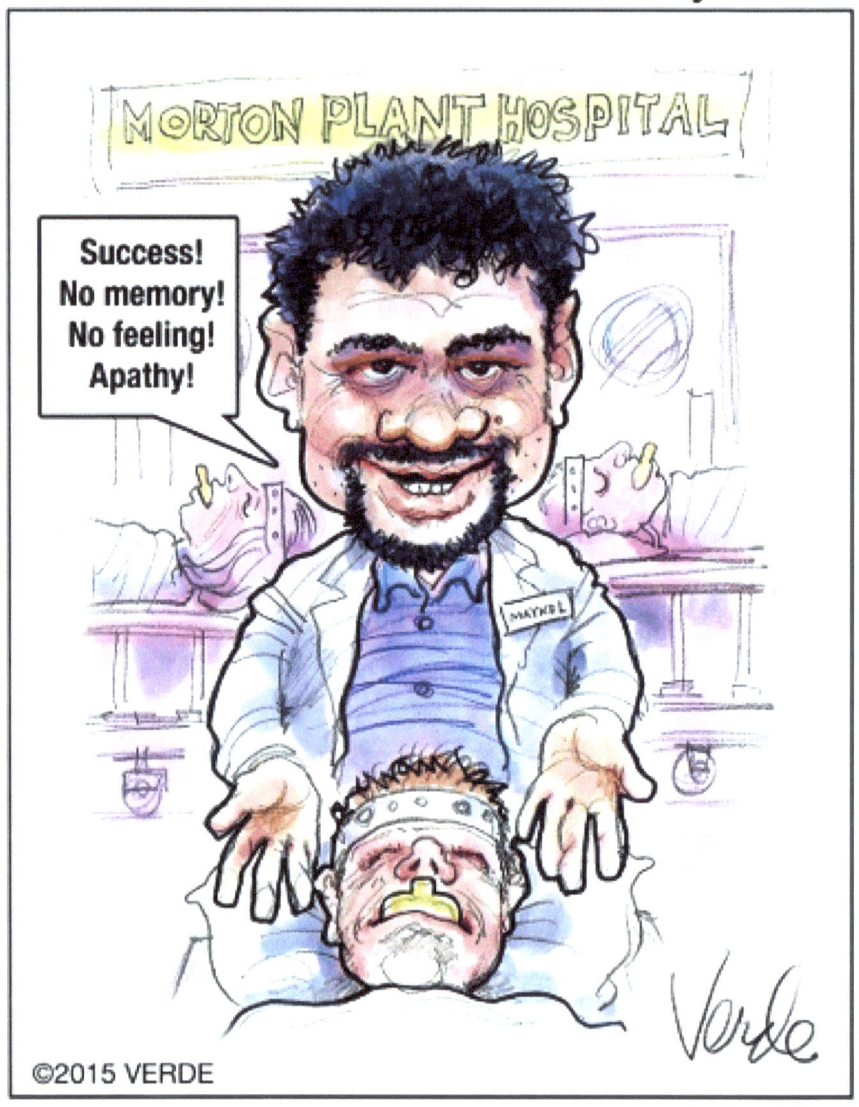

Yes, psychiatrists still do shock treatment.

Yikes! The Psychs! by Horst Dubiel

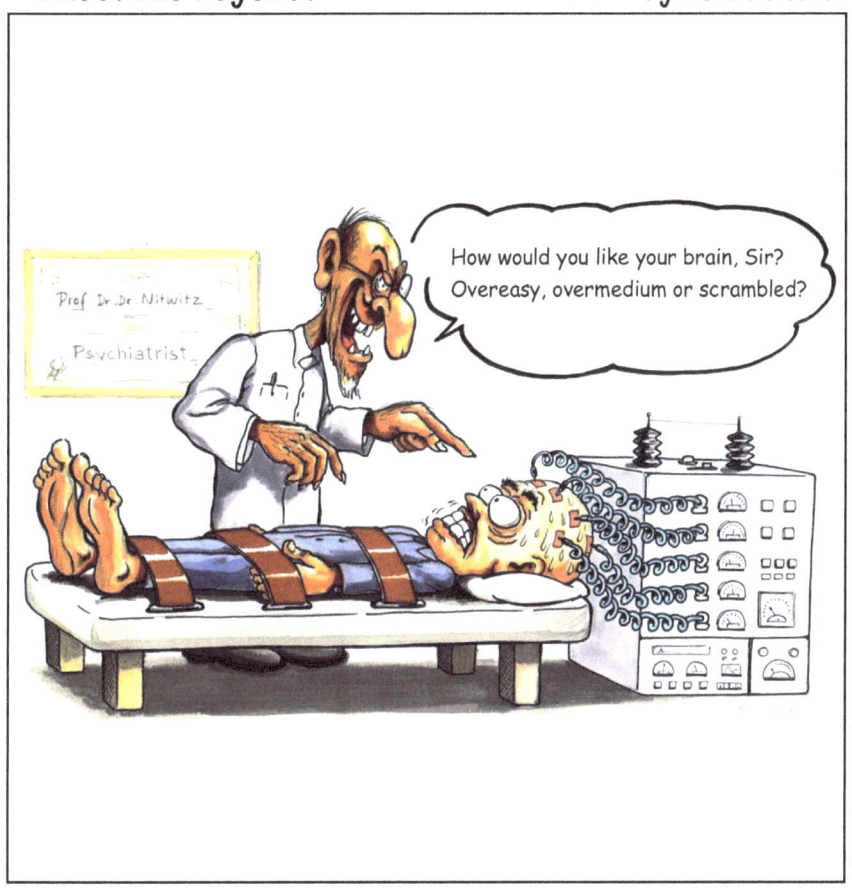

The "Shrink" Tank   by Verde

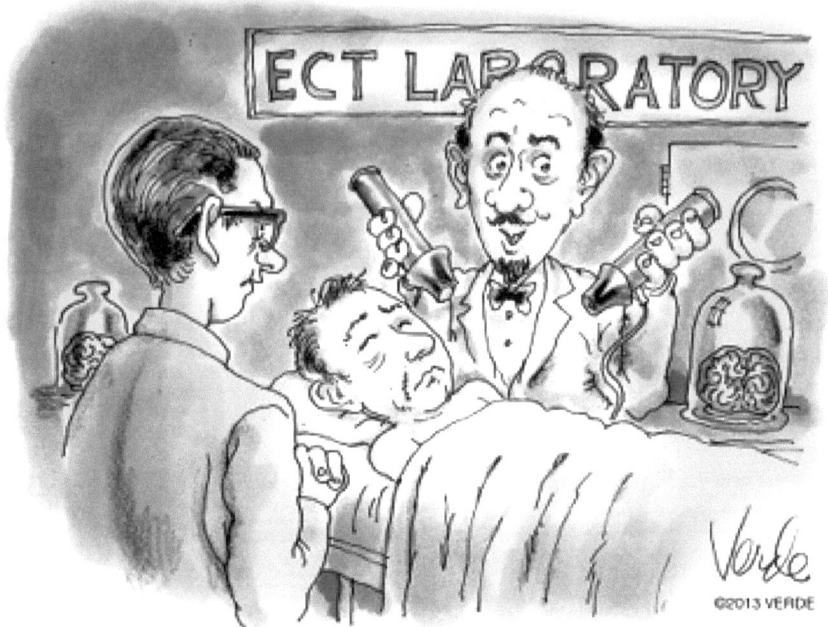

"You may enjoy watching a foot quiver like I do."

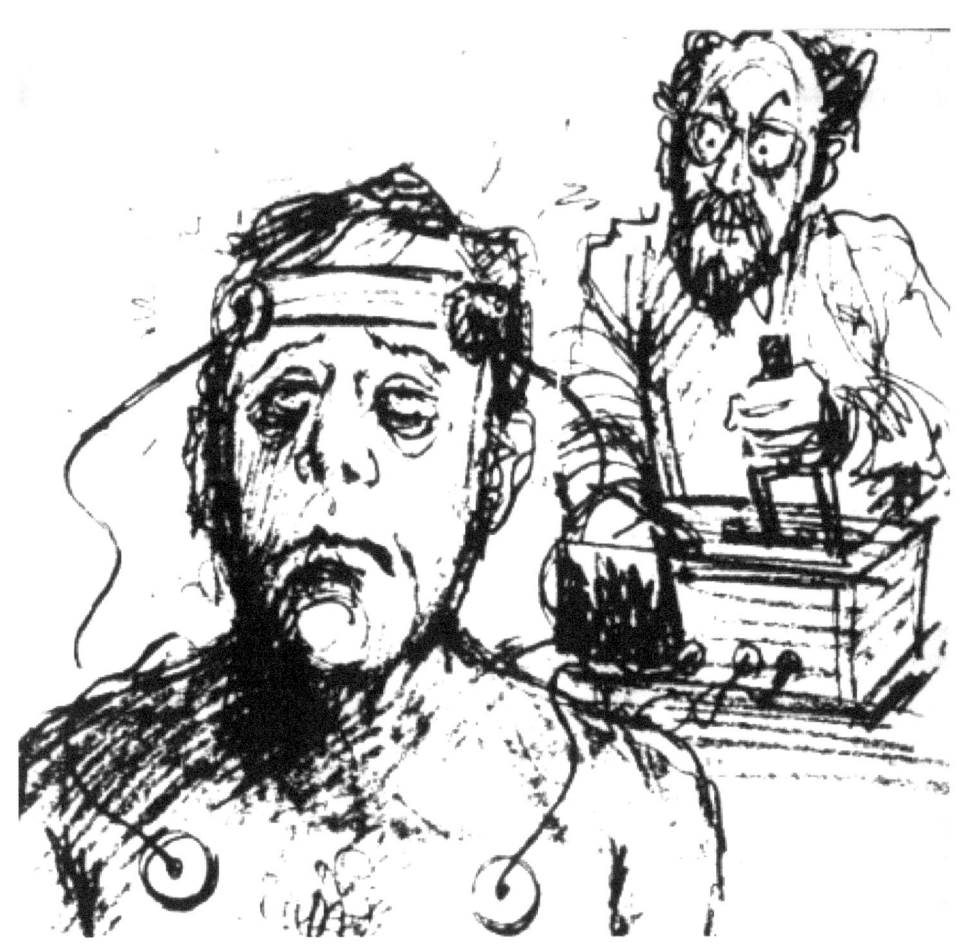

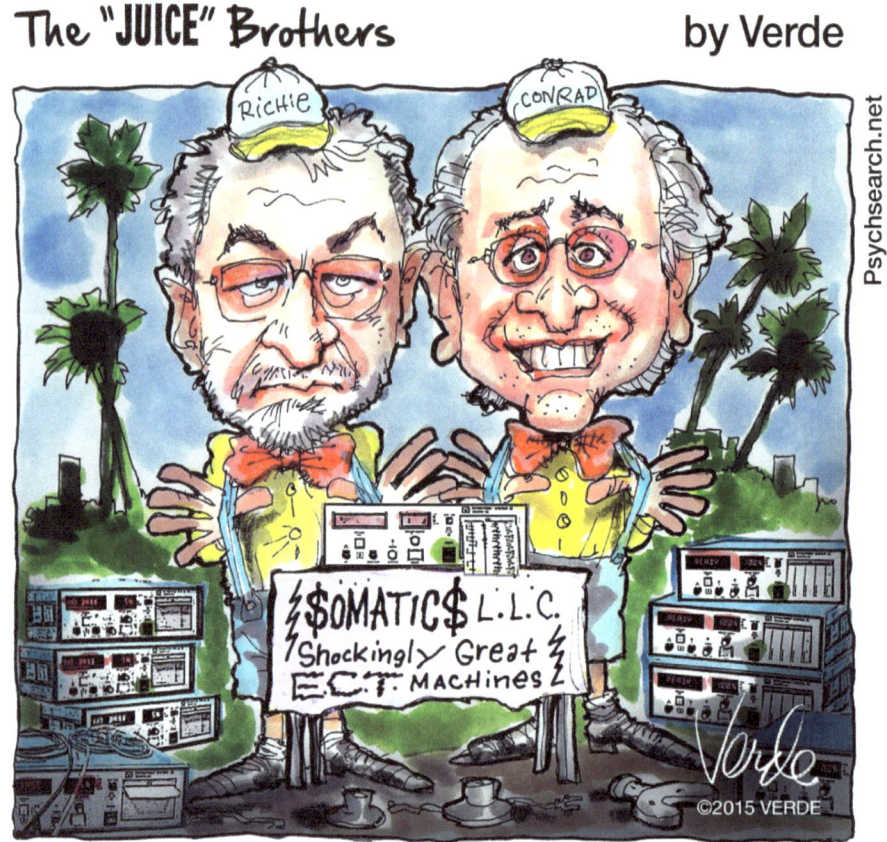

"Abrams and Swartz, now Open for Business in sunny Florida!"

SEXUAL MISCONDUCT

"Sexual misconduct is particularly damaging to the reputation of psychiatry because the damages to patients which result are mental and emotional in nature. If psychiatry loses the confidence of society, its ability to pursue its mission will be damaged."

American Psychiatric Association
Approved by the Board of Trustees
March 1993

The "Shrink" Tank

by Verde

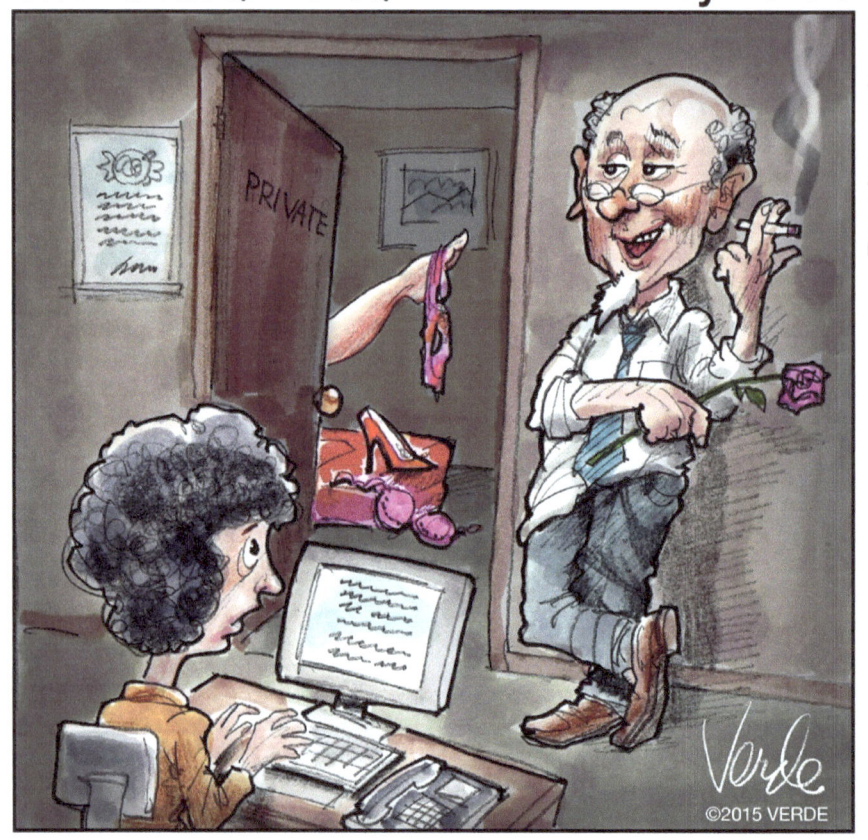

"Cancel all appointments ... my patient is calling."

Psych-Sex   by Verde

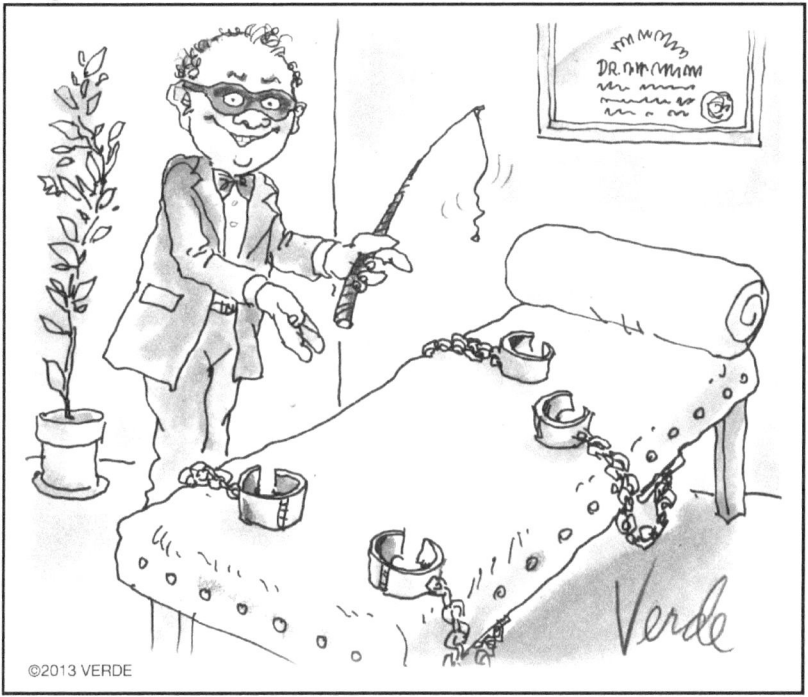

Psychs

by Kramer & Brown

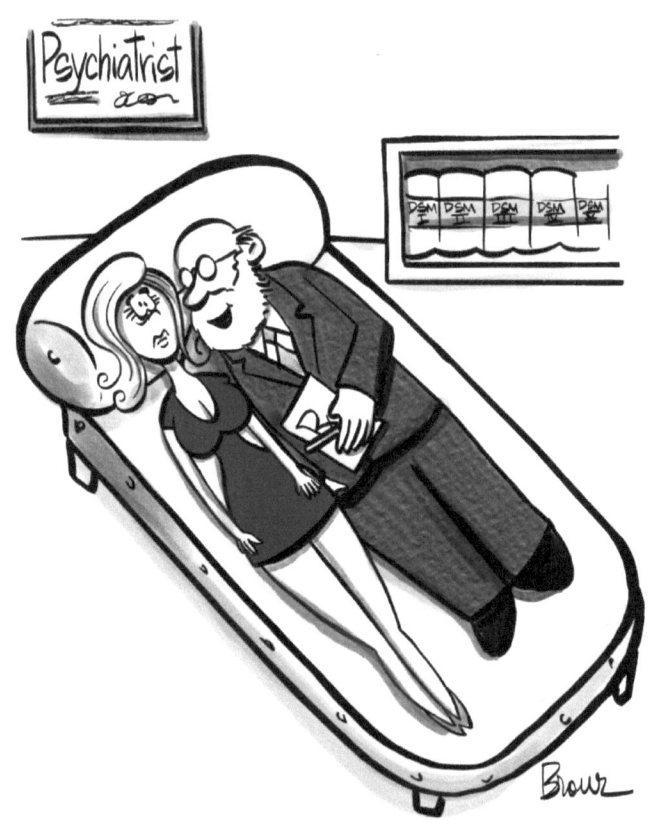

"Tell me more about your fear of intimacy."

NO SCIENCE

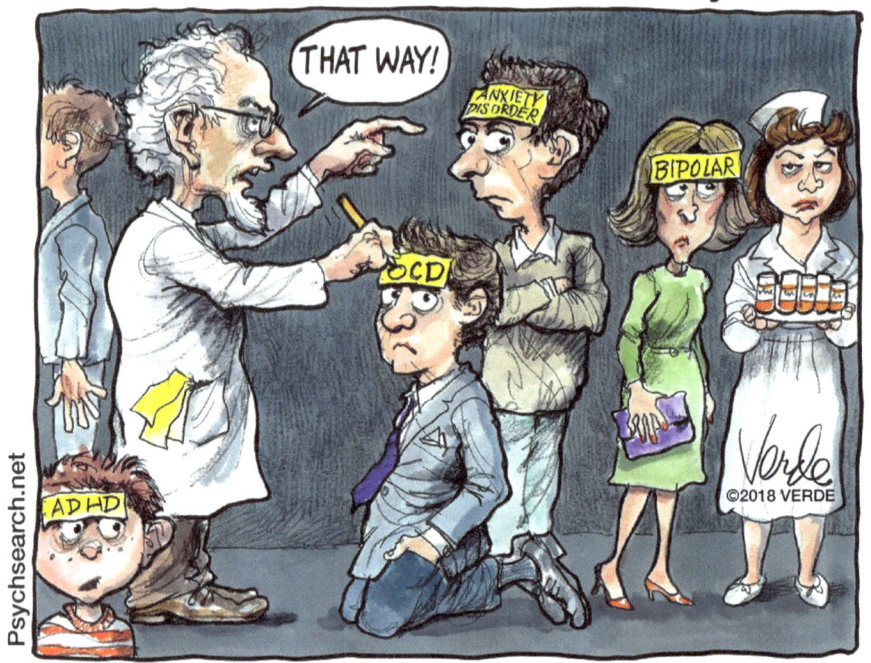

Psychiatry: The "Church" of the Holy Label

Psychs

by Kramer & Brown

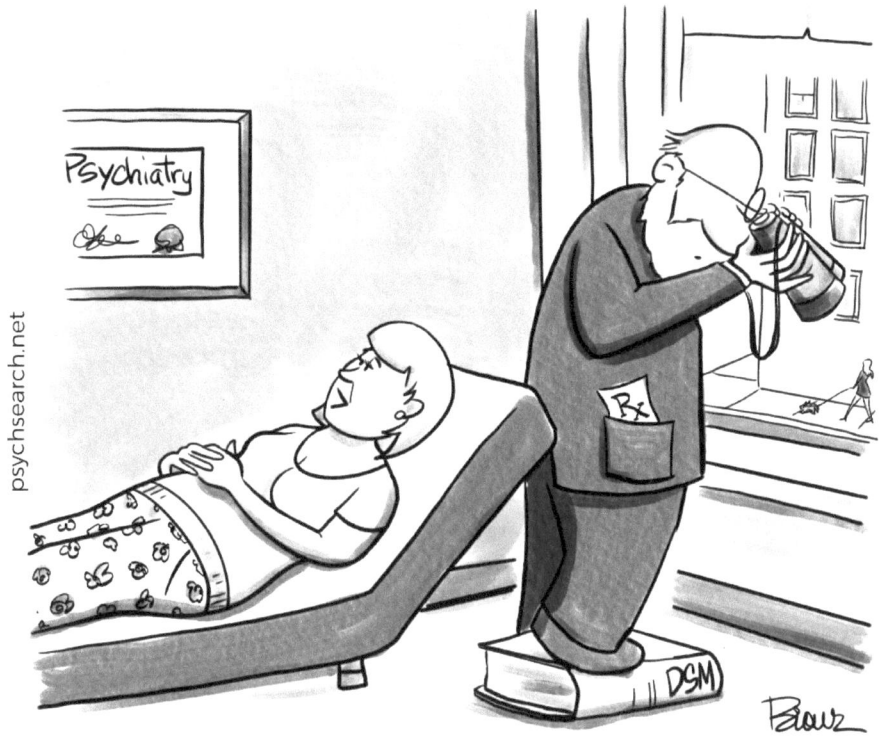

"No one ever pays attention to me."

Psychs

by Kramer & Brown

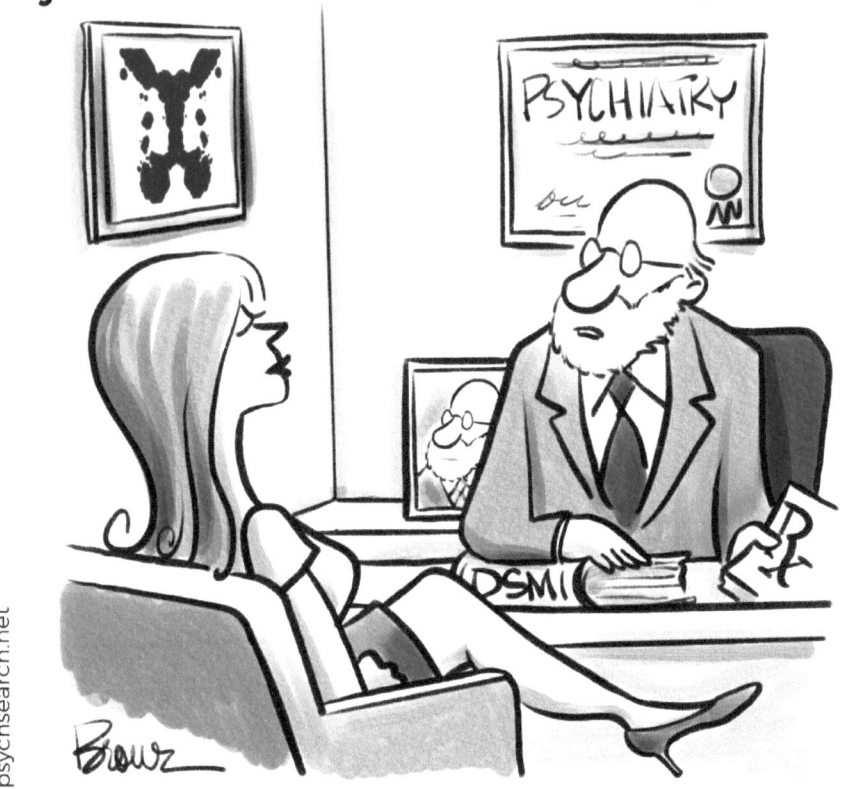

"Lab tests? We don't need no stinkin' lab tests! Just by looking at you I can see you have a chemical imbalance!"

Psychs

by Kramer & Brown

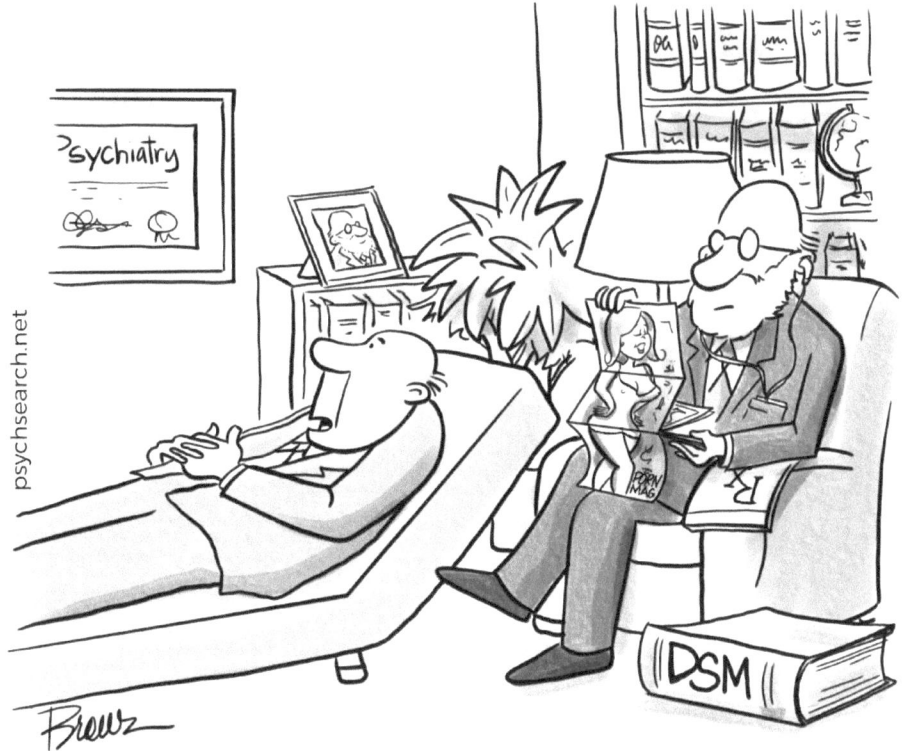

"No one ever listens to me."

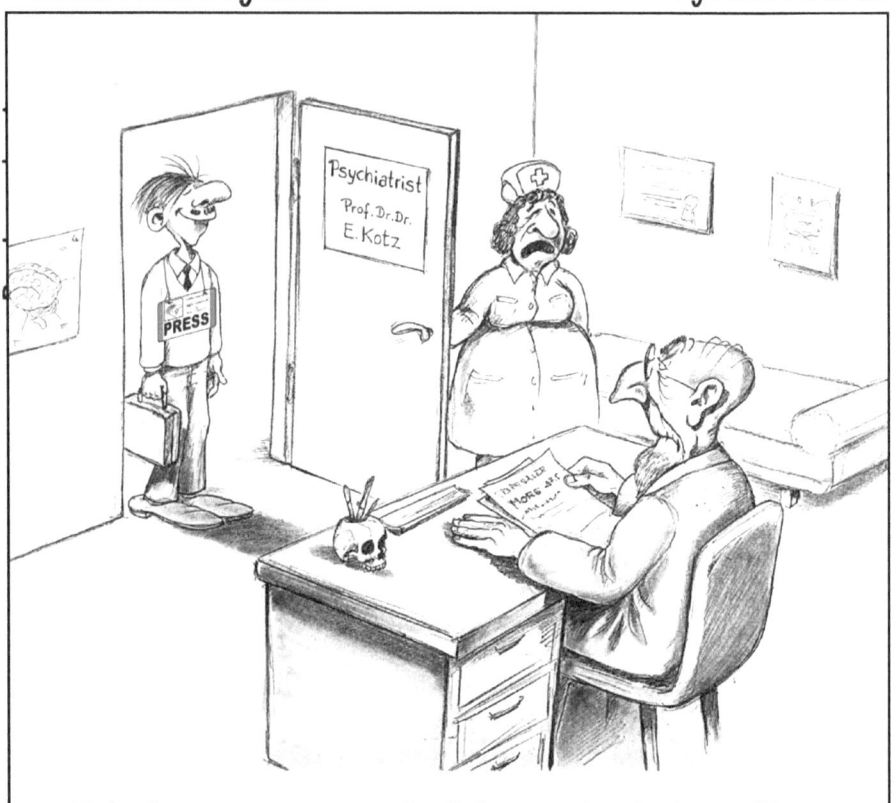

56

Psychsearch.net

Shrink Tank

by Verde

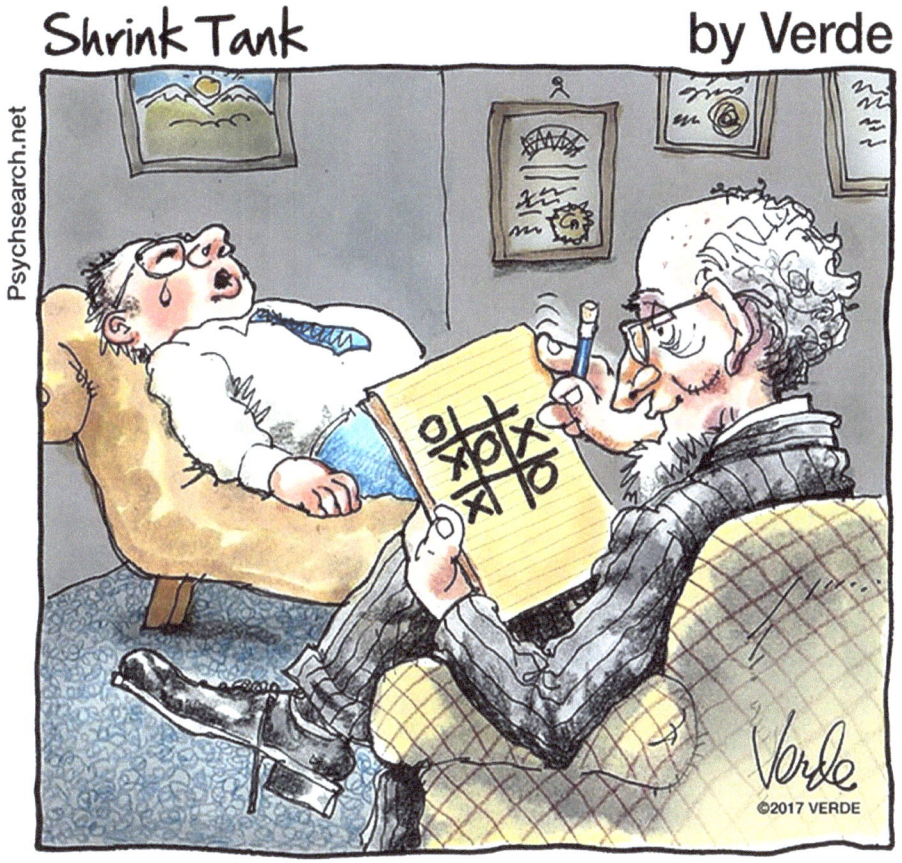

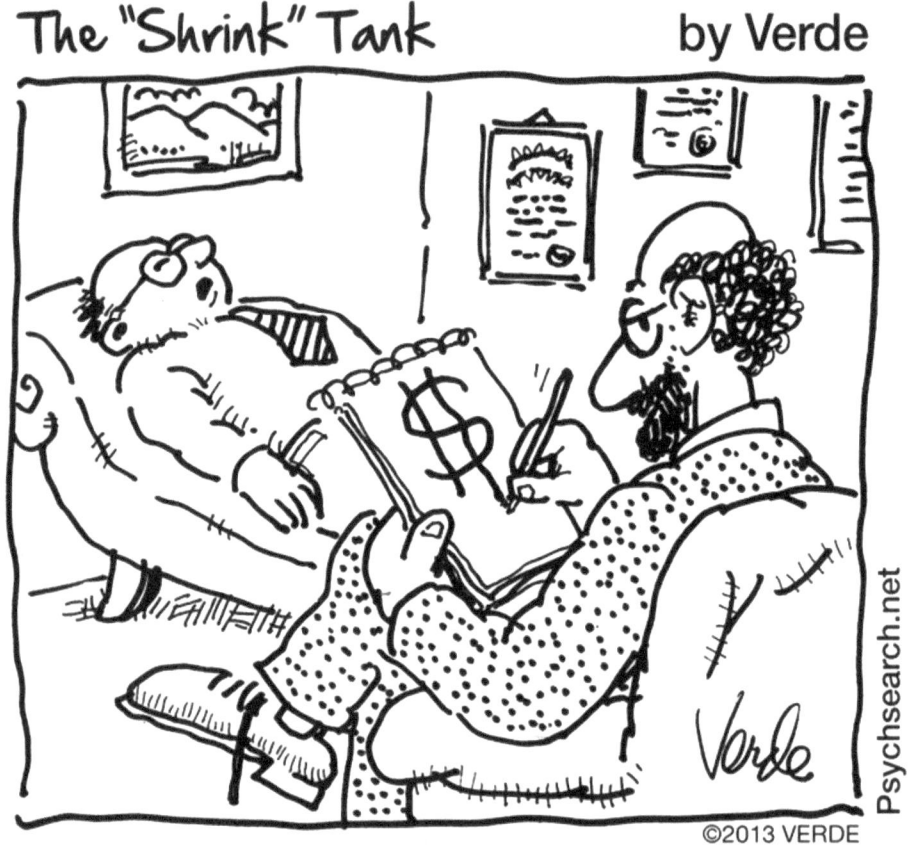

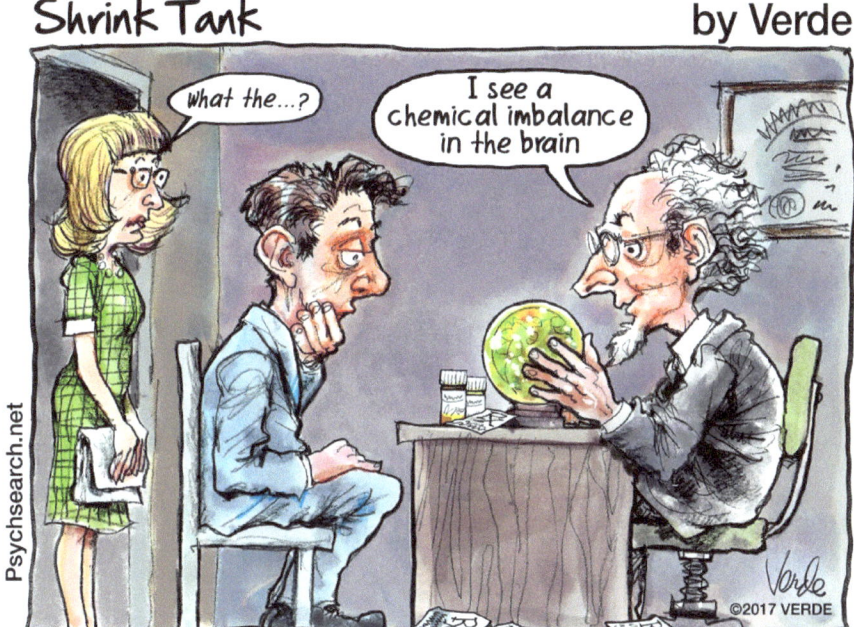

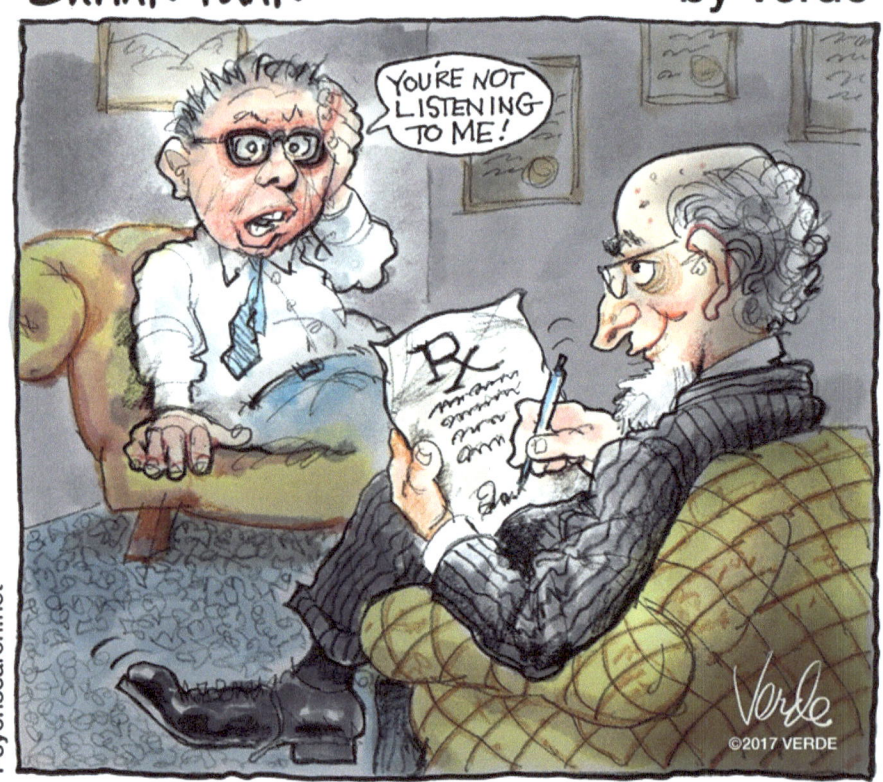

"Pardon—I was just making some notes."

PSYCH DRUGS
PSYCHIATRIC ~~TOOLS~~ WEAPONS

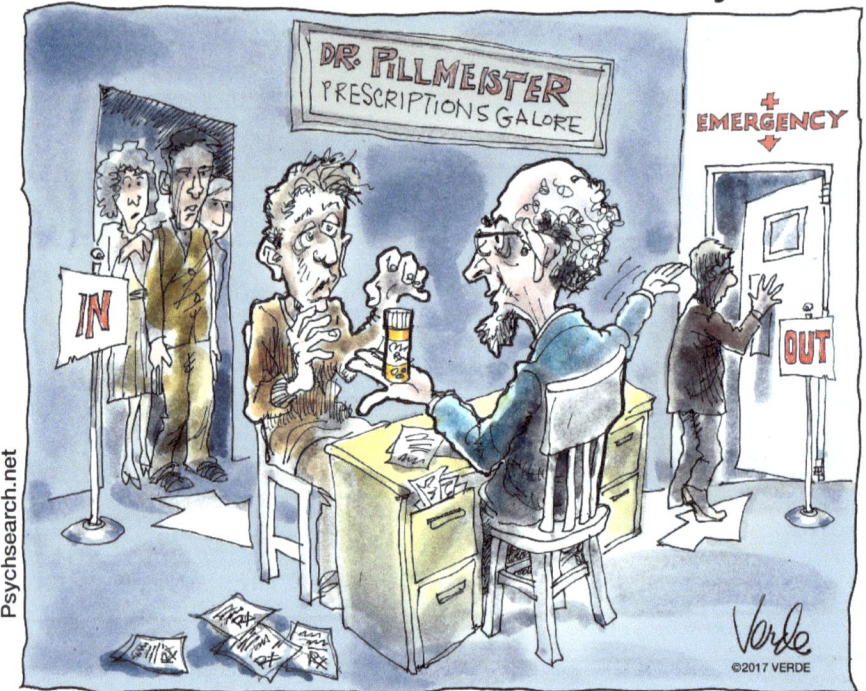

Pill Mill

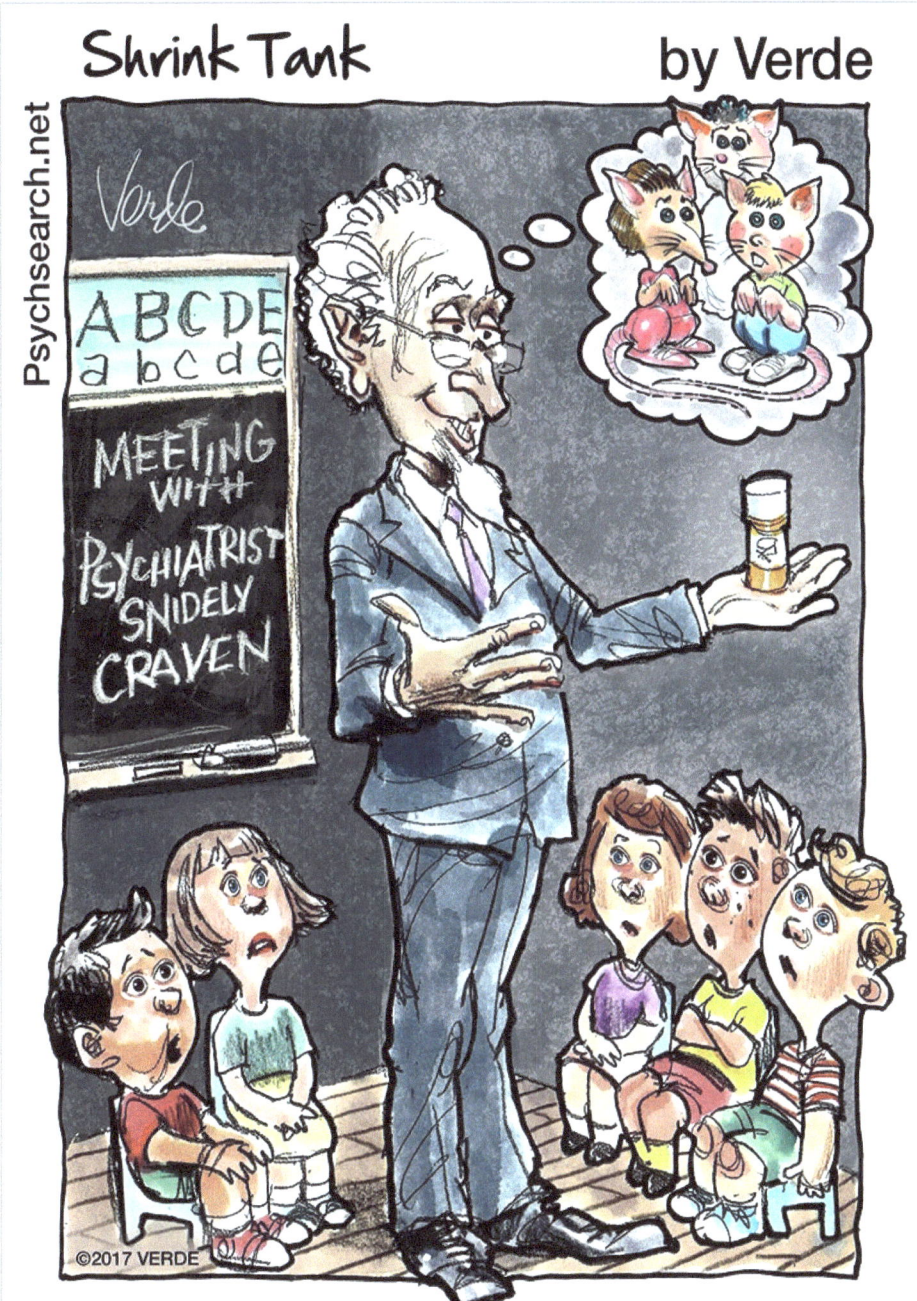

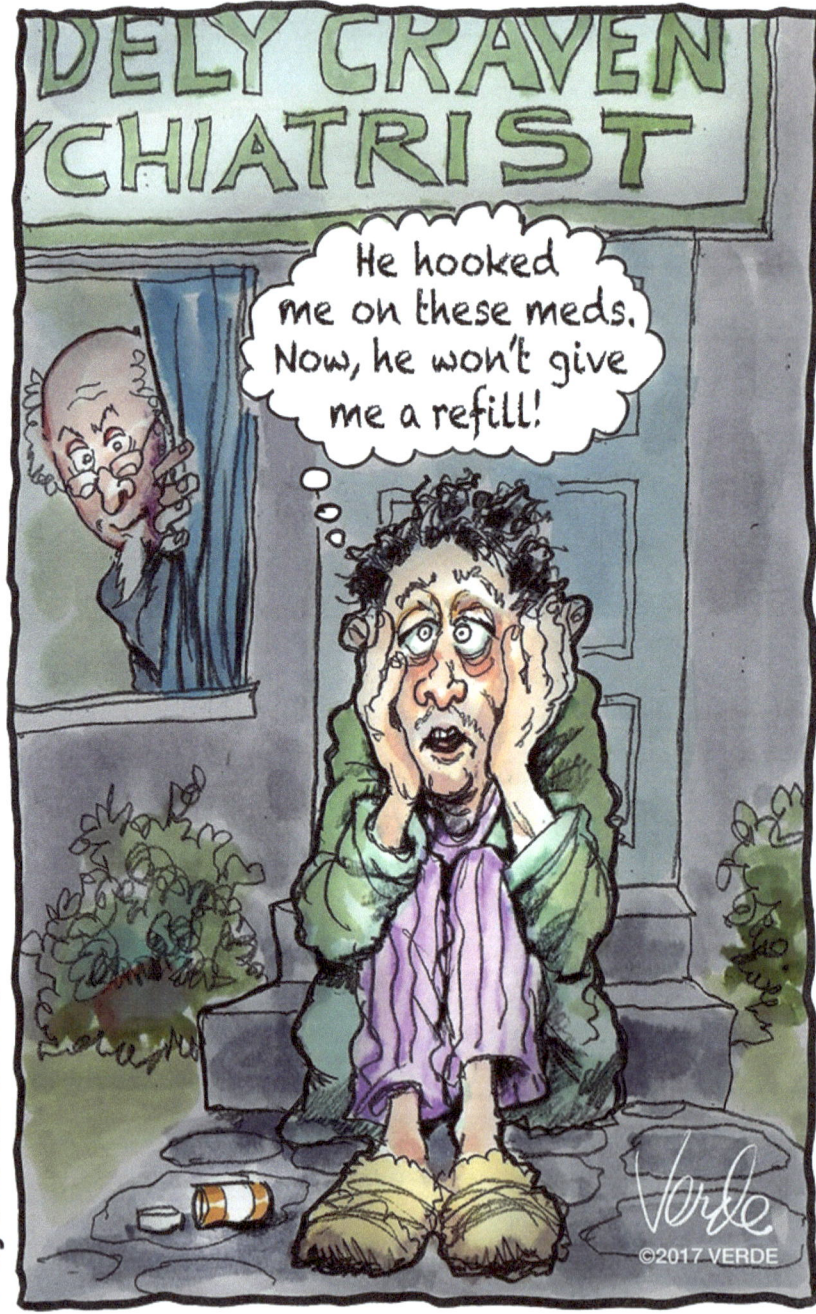

Psychs

by Kramer & Brown

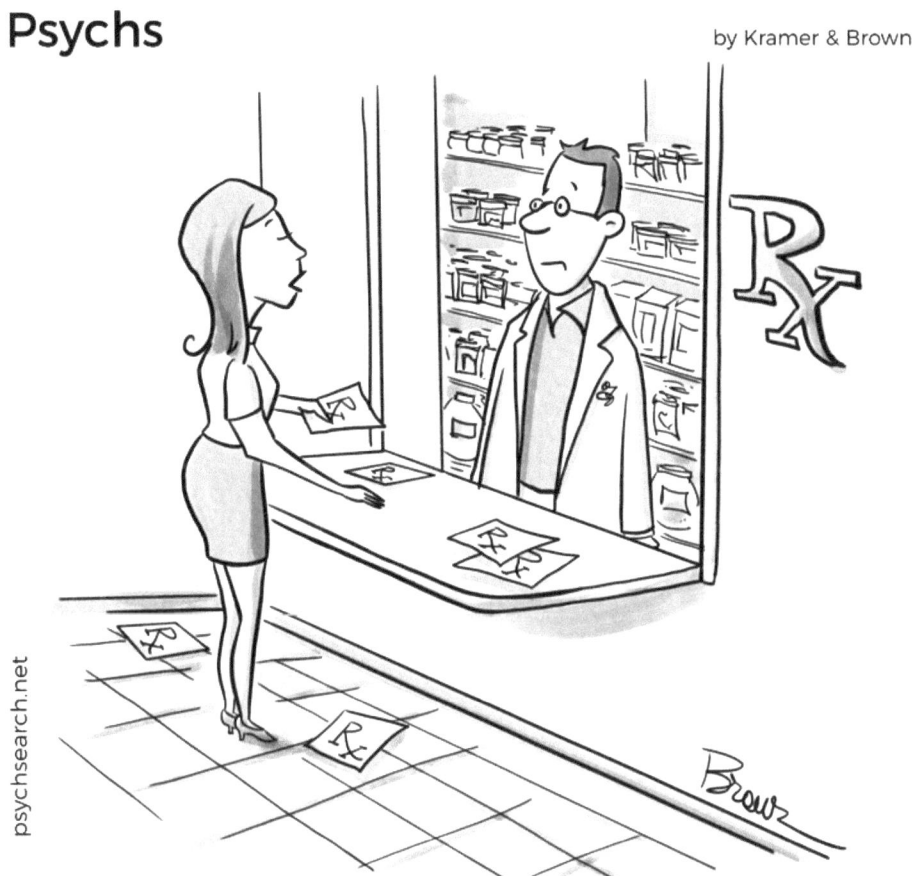

"So sorry! My psychiatrist has Obsessive Prescribing Disorder!"

Psychs

by Kramer & Brown

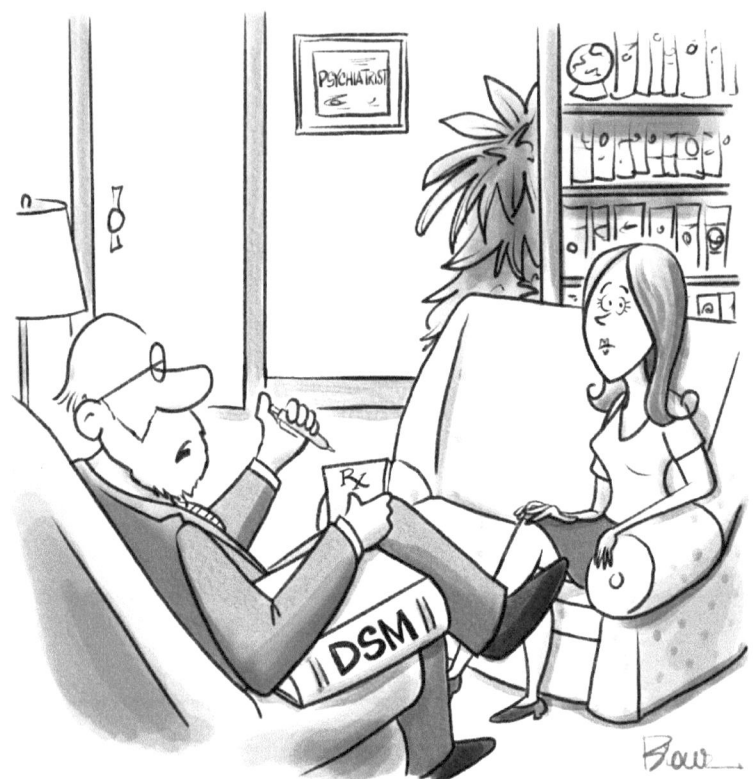

"I don't have time to listen to all that.
*I only do what we call in the biz, **Medication Management***
By the way, do you have any plans for this evening?"

Yikes! The Psychs!   by Horst Dubiel

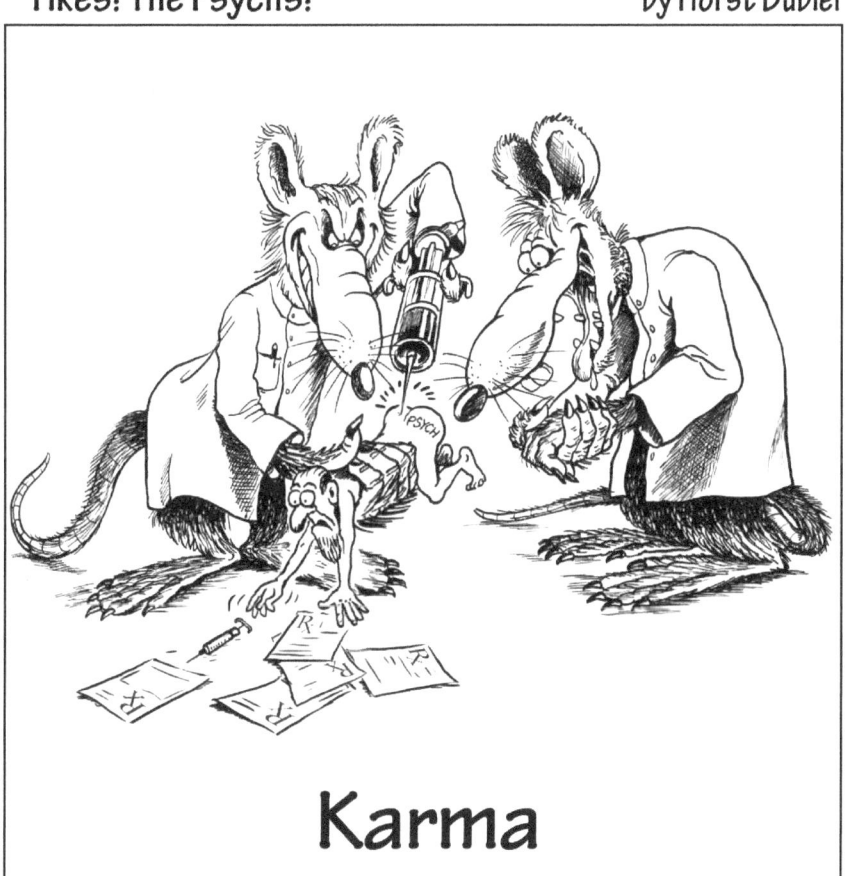

PsychSearch.net

Karma

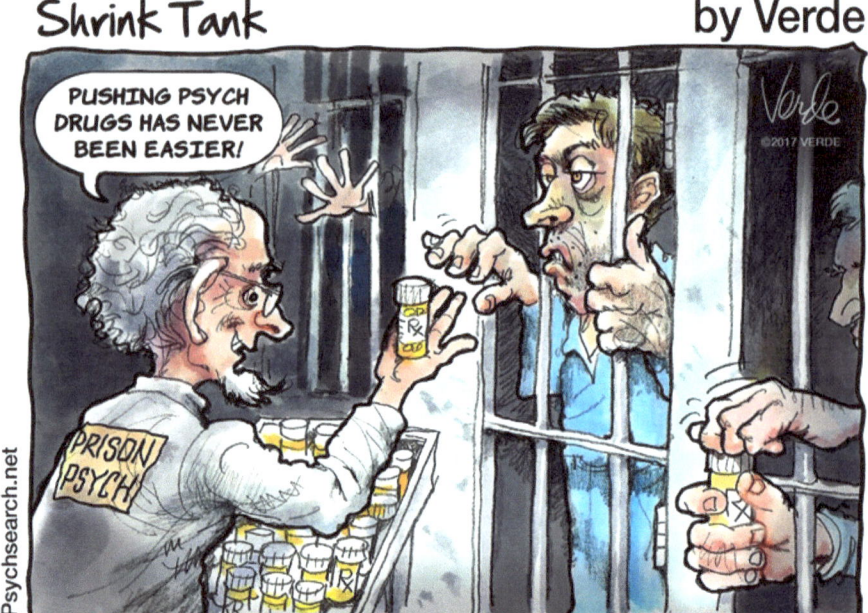

"Jails and prisons—mental asylums of the 21st century."

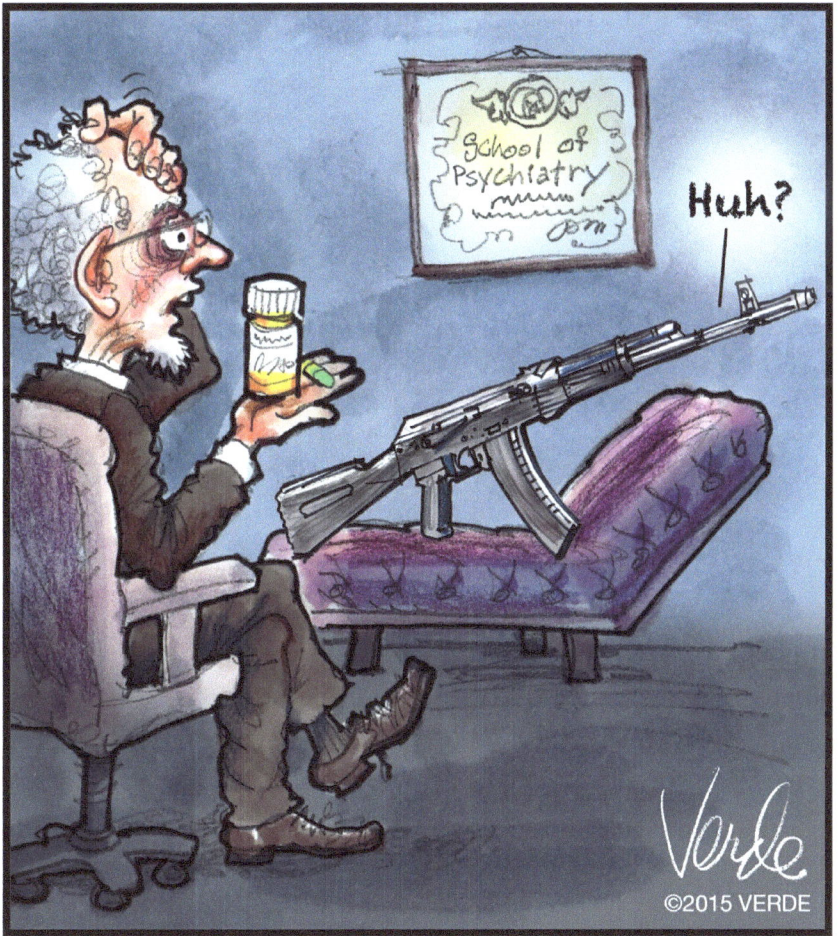

"Those thoughts of killing all those innocent people came from taking two pills... let's try one."

Shrink Tank

by Verde

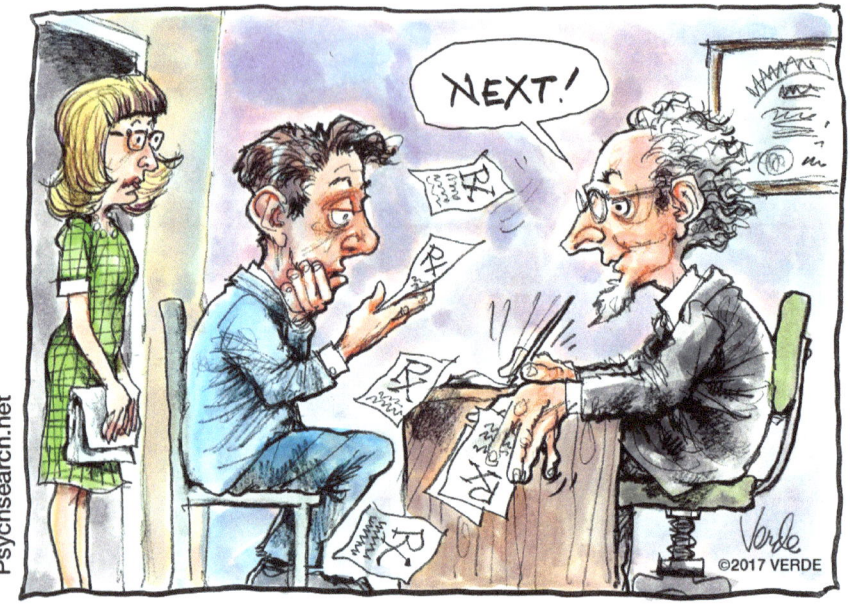

"Psychiatrists suffer from Obsessive Prescribing Disorder."

The "Shrink" Tank
by Verde

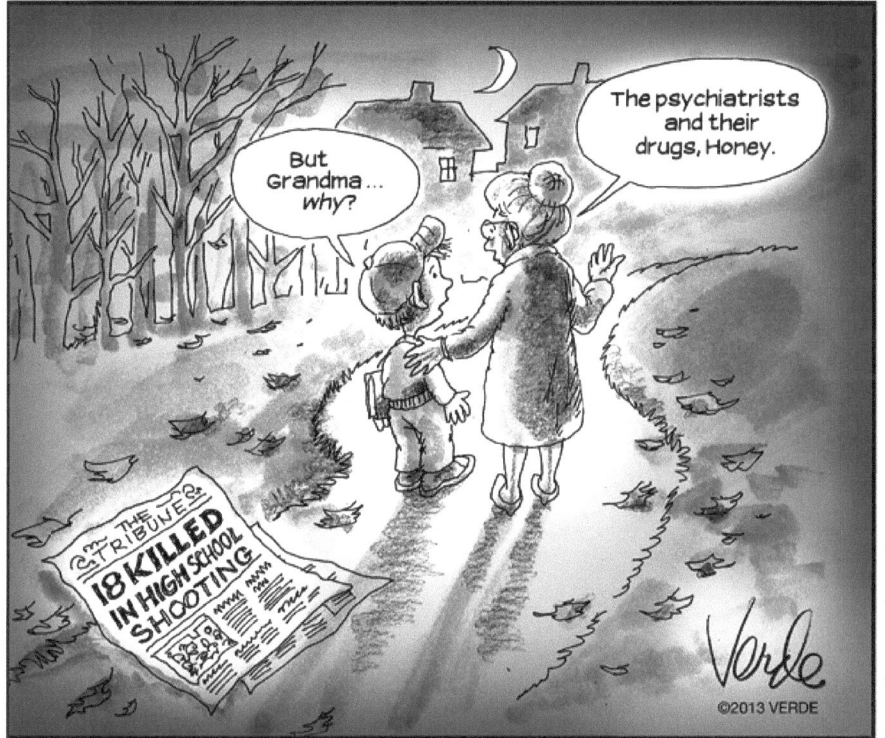

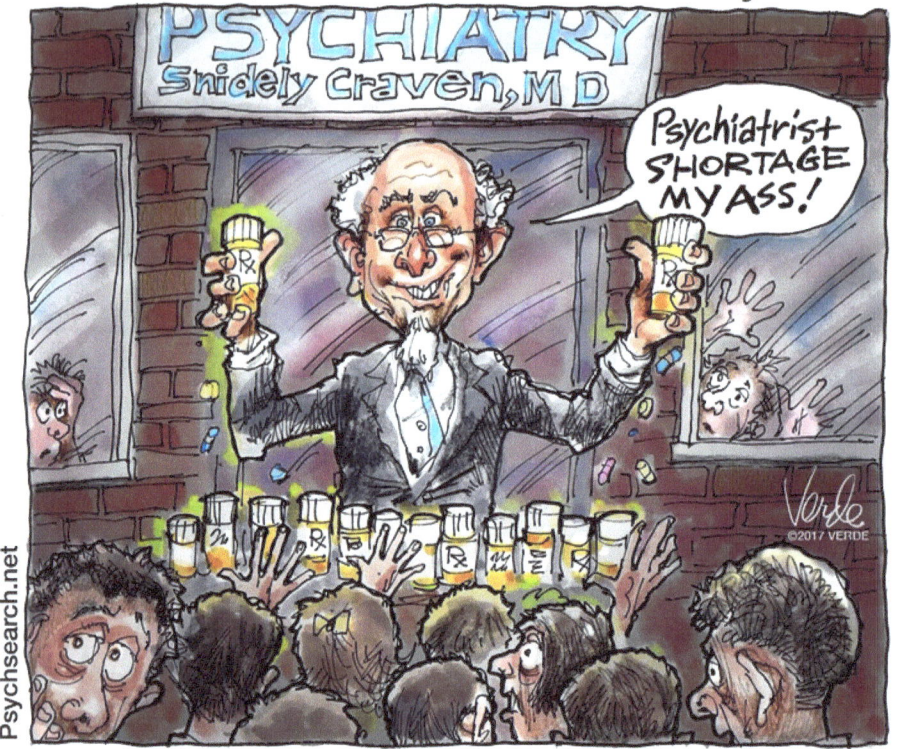

"I'll drug every one of y'all!"

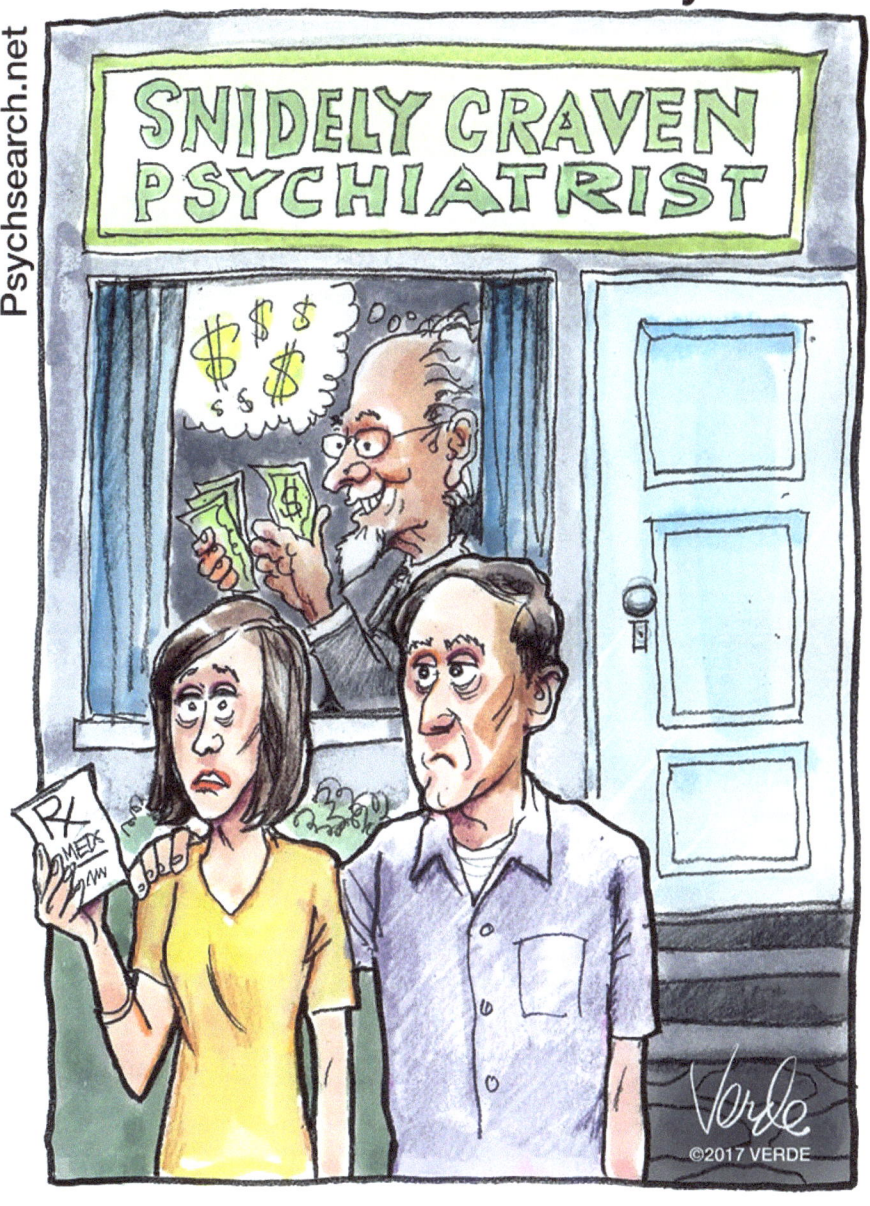

Shrink Tank
by Verde

Psychsearch.net

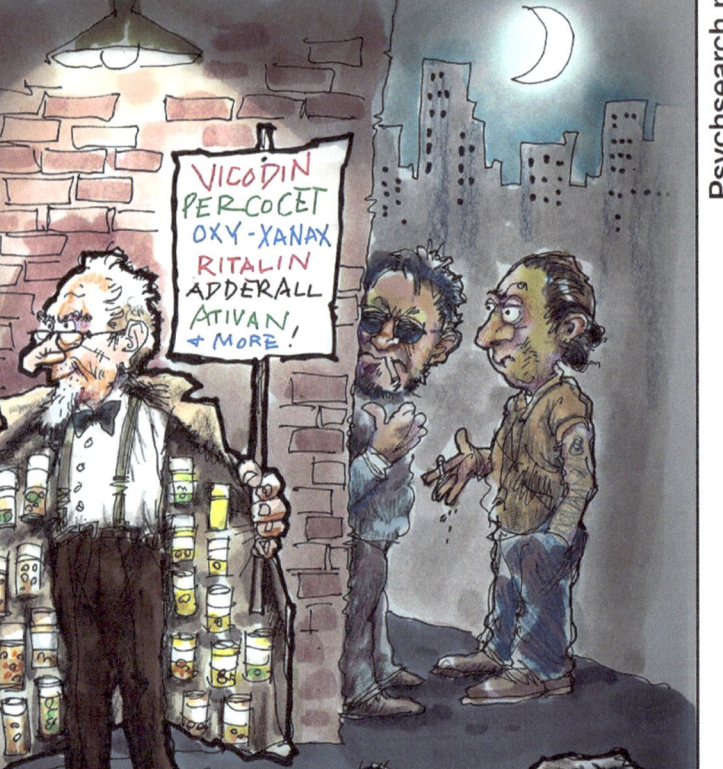

"These Psychs have been moving in on our territory lately."

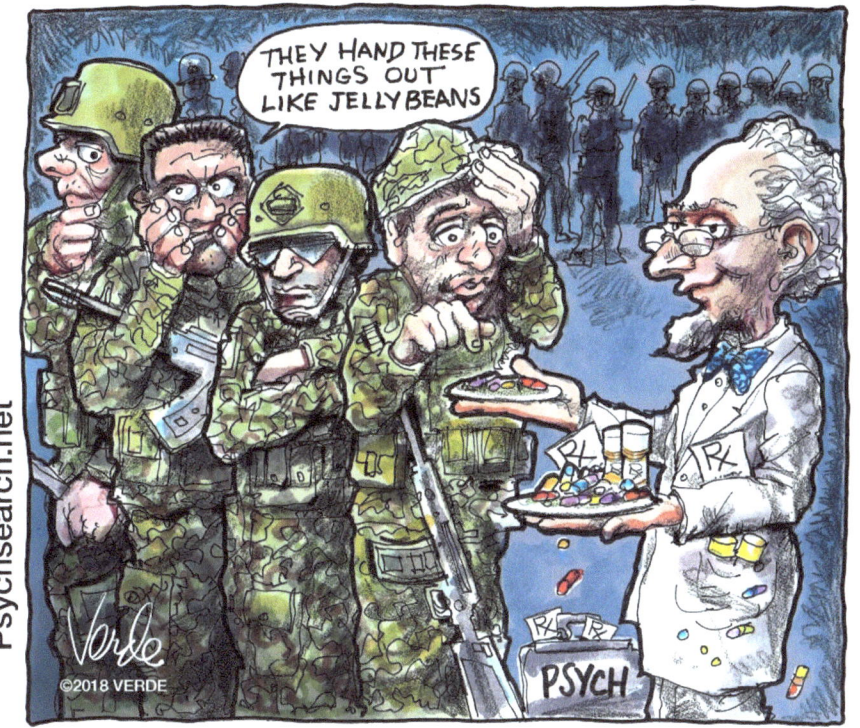

"Baffling Rise in Suicides Plagues U.S. Military"
— The New York Times

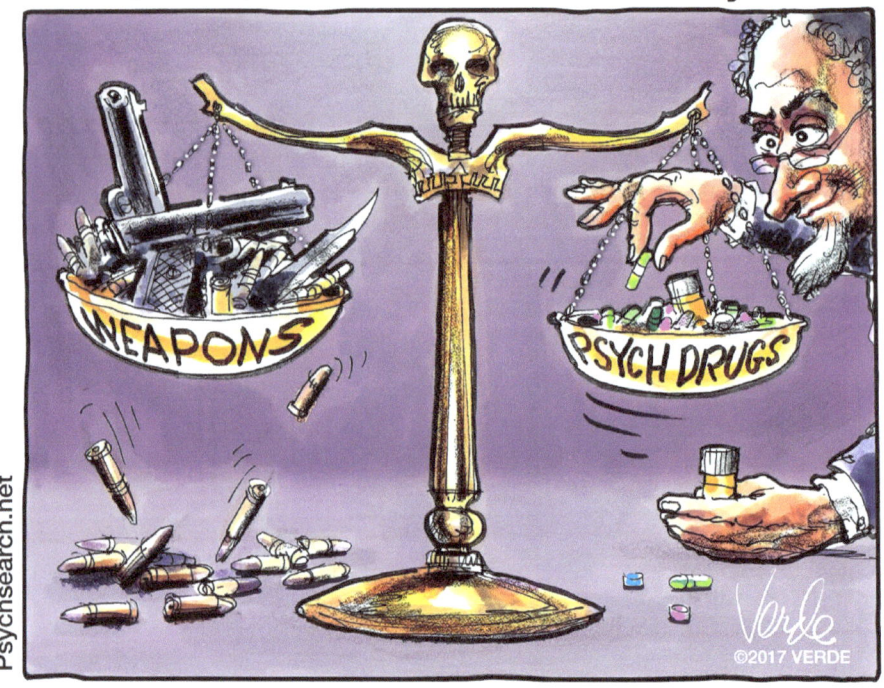

Weighing Destruction

Yikes! The Psychs! by Horst Dubiel

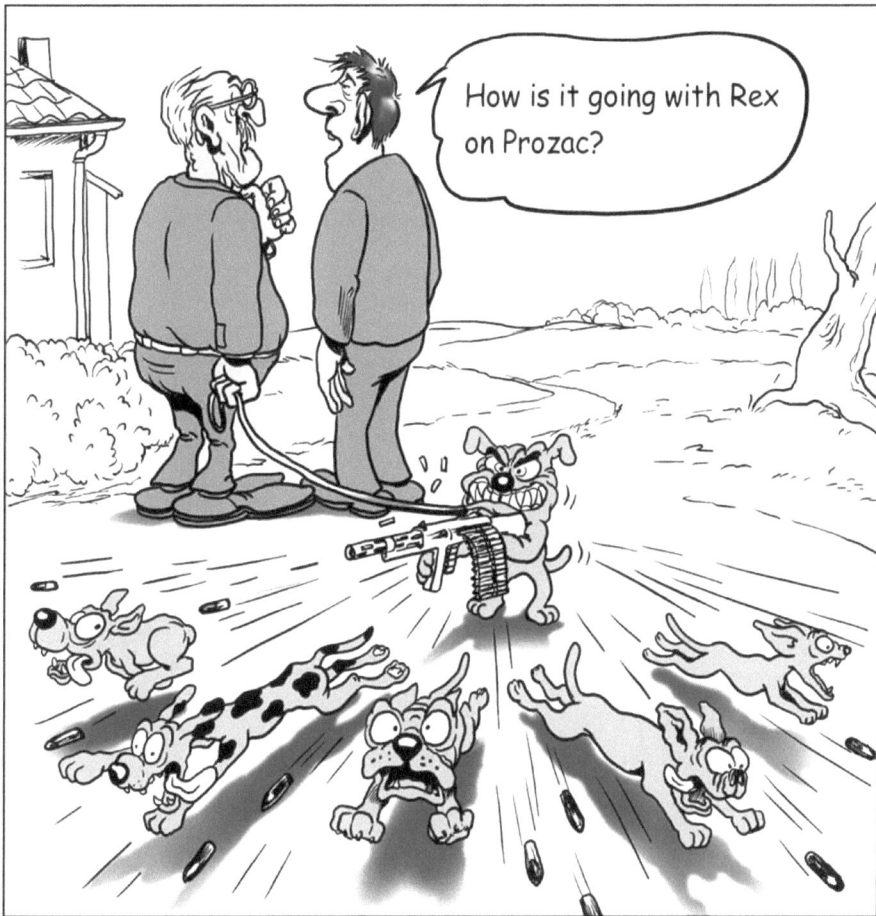

Yikes! The Psychs!   by Horst Dubiel

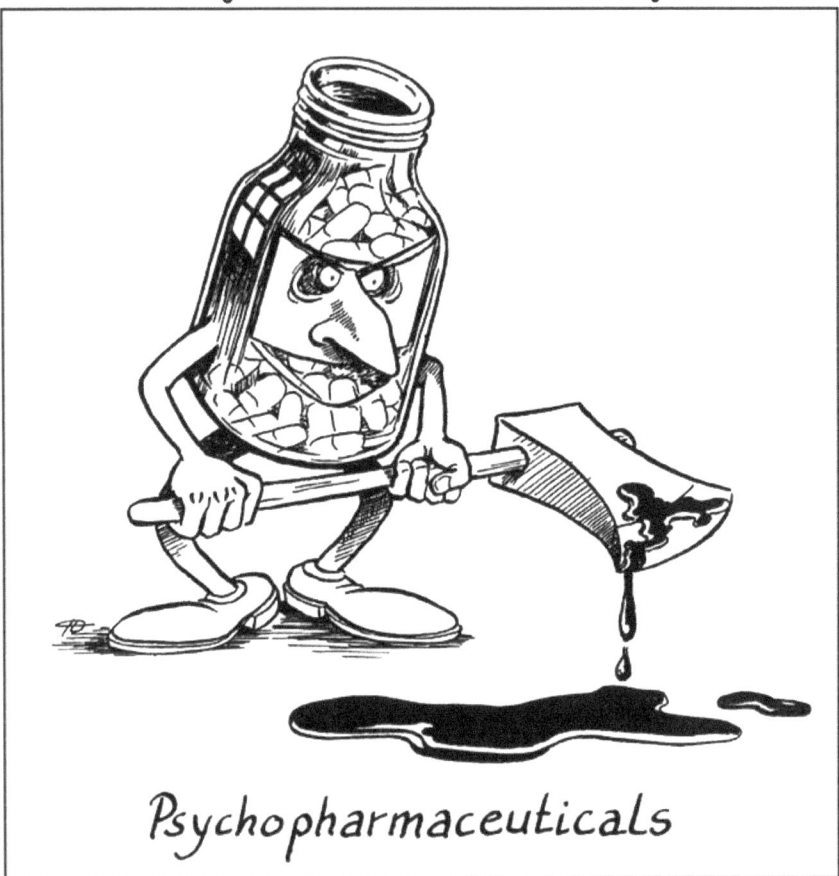

Psychopharmaceuticals

PsychSearch.net

OTHER PRACTICES

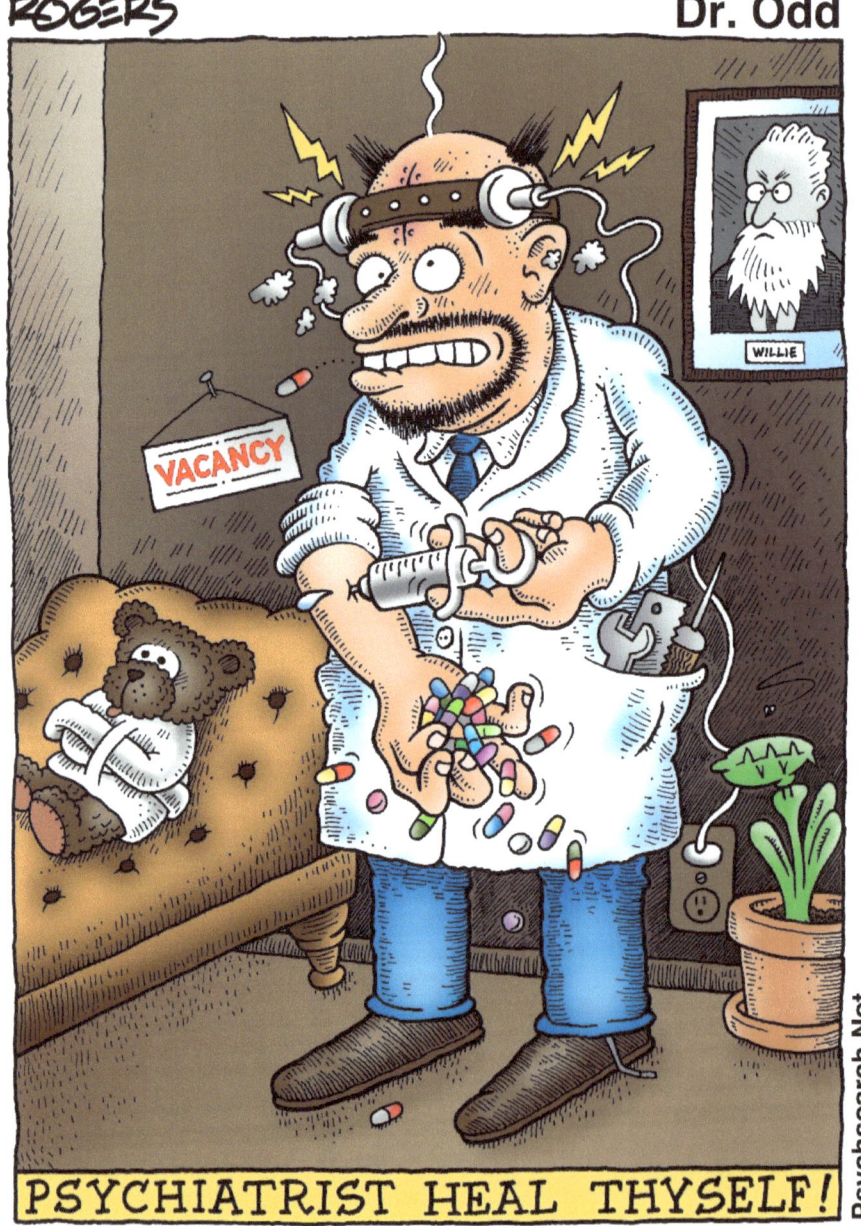

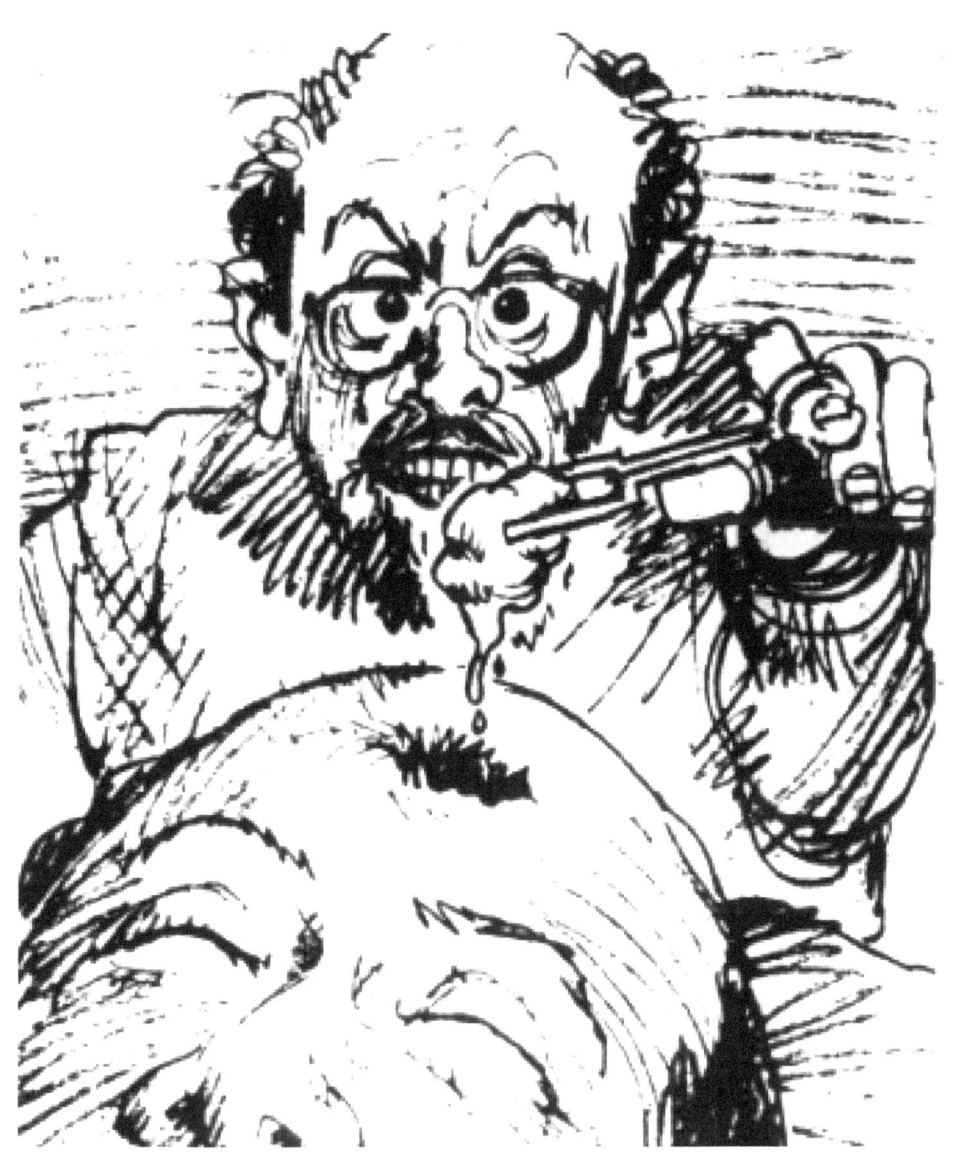

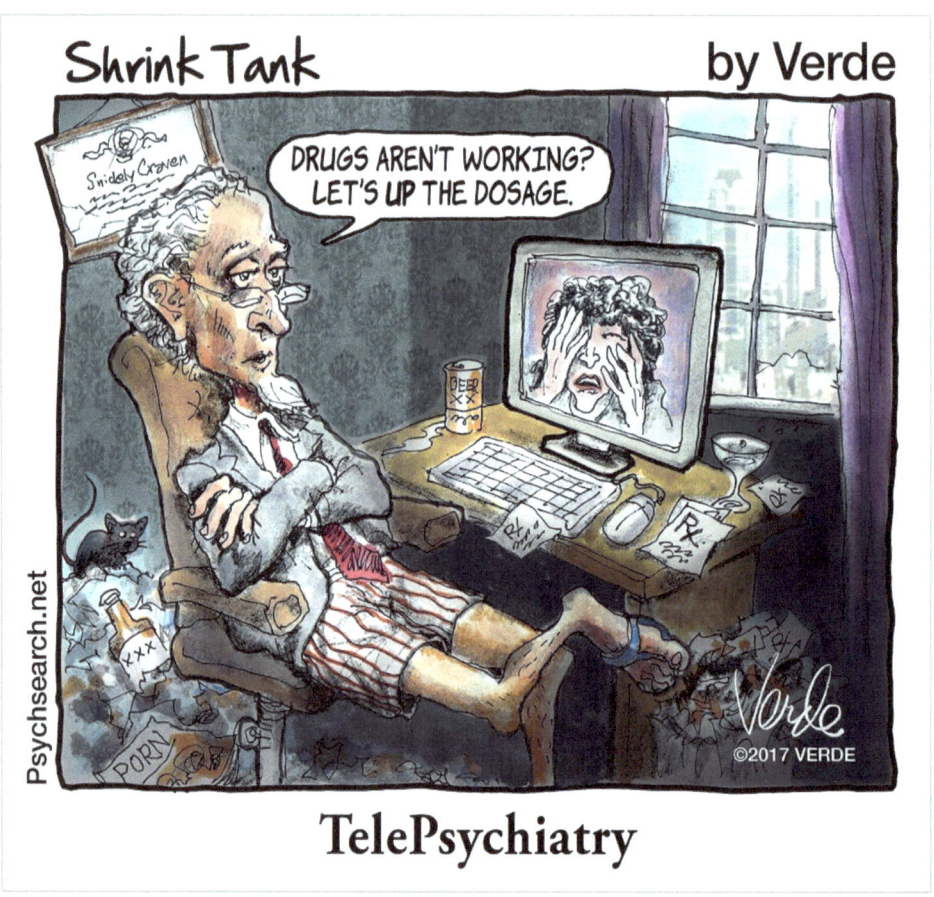

The "Tools" of Psychiatry

by Verde

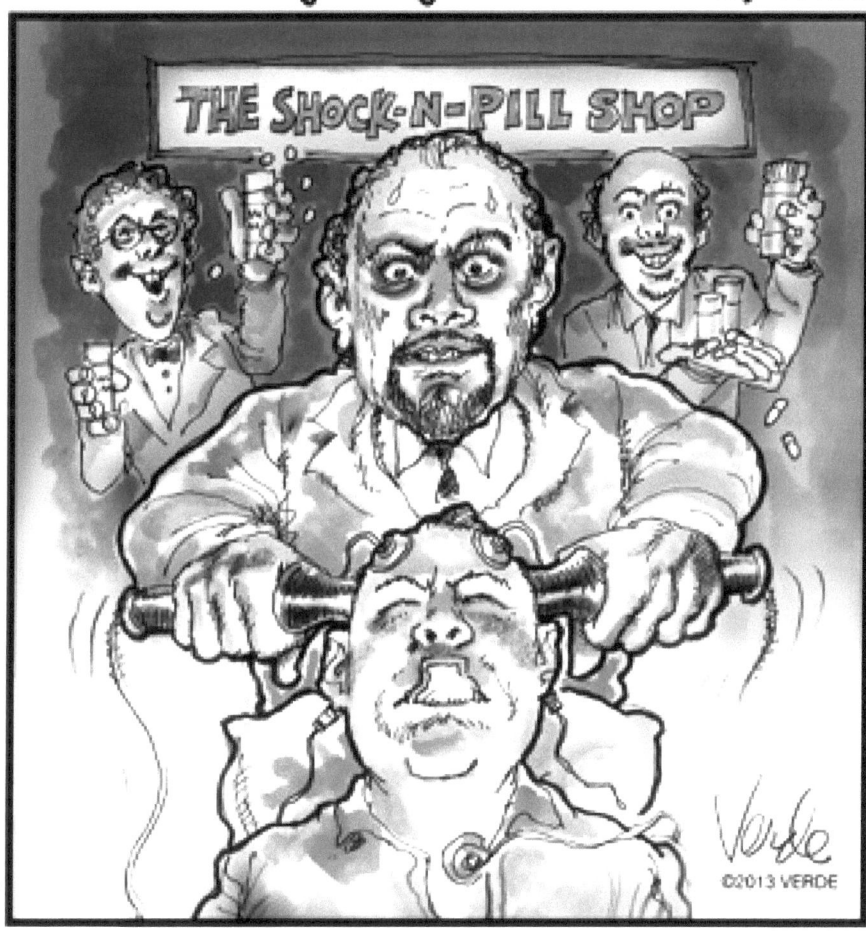

THE SHOCK-N-PILL SHOP

©2013 VERDE

Psychsearch.net

OFF THE WALL

Shrink Tank
by Verde

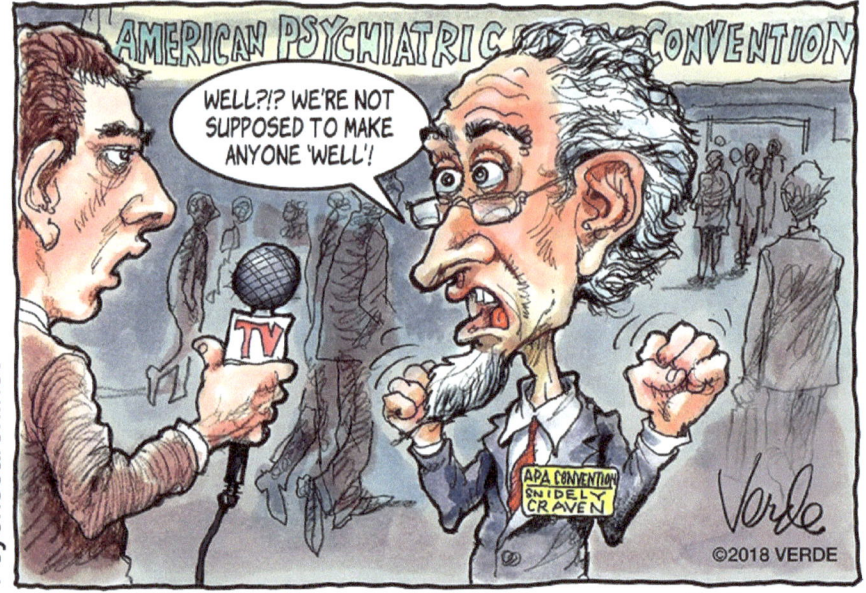

"Have you ever made anyone *well*?"

Yikes! The Psychs!　　　　　　　　　　　by Horst Dubiel

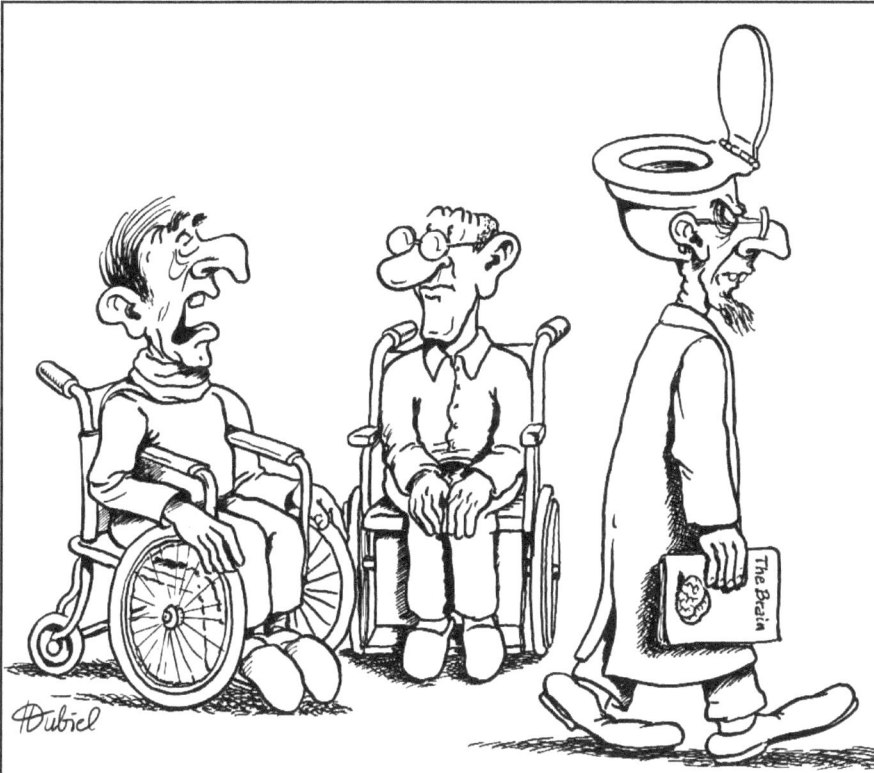

You know, I have often wondered what actually goes on in the head of a psychiatrist.

PsychSearch.net

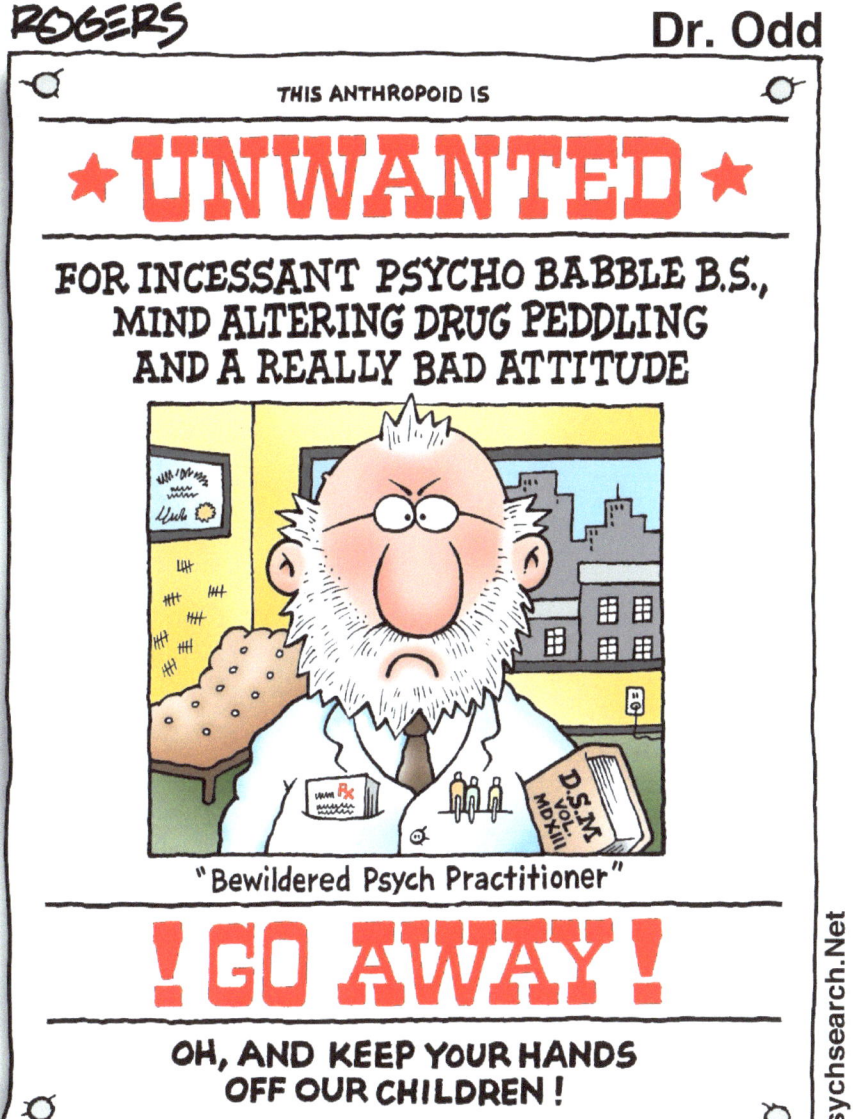

Yikes! The Psychs! by Horst Dubiel

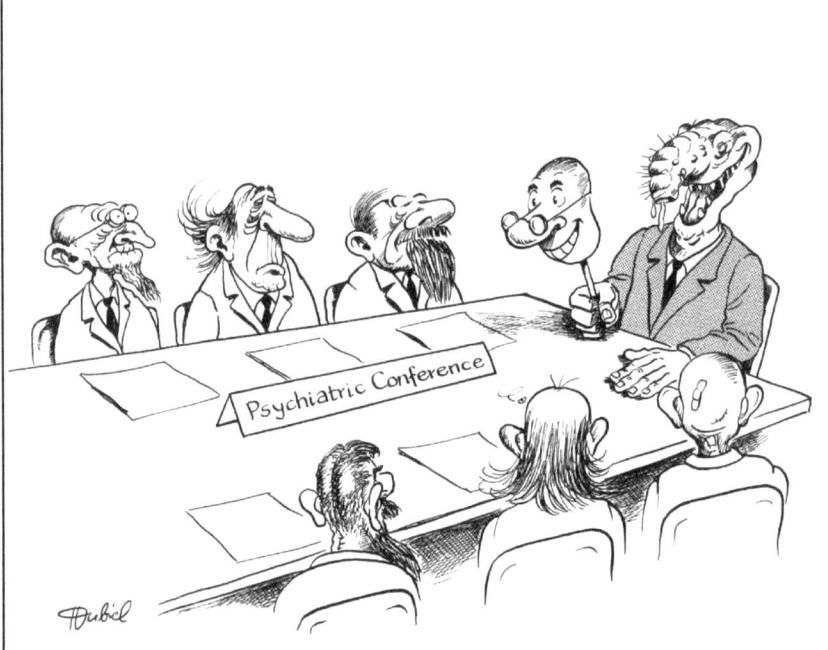

Finally, we're all alone – off with the masks!

PsychSearch.net

Yikes! The Psychs!   by Horst Dubiel

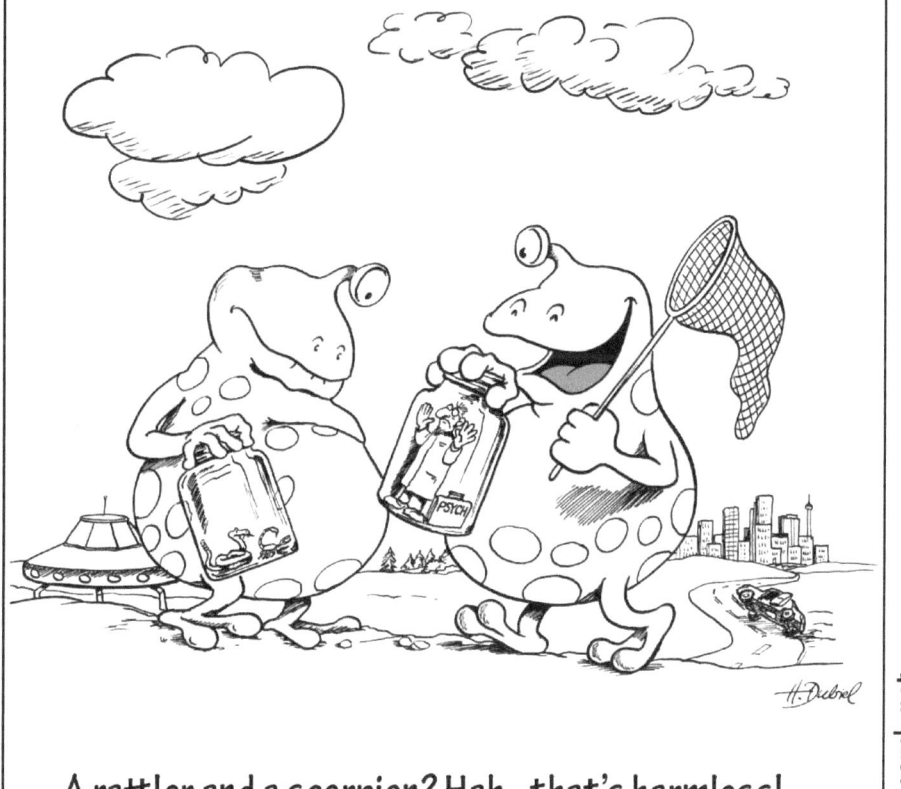

A rattler and a scorpion? Hah - that's harmless!
Look what I have got!

Psychs

by Kramer & Brown

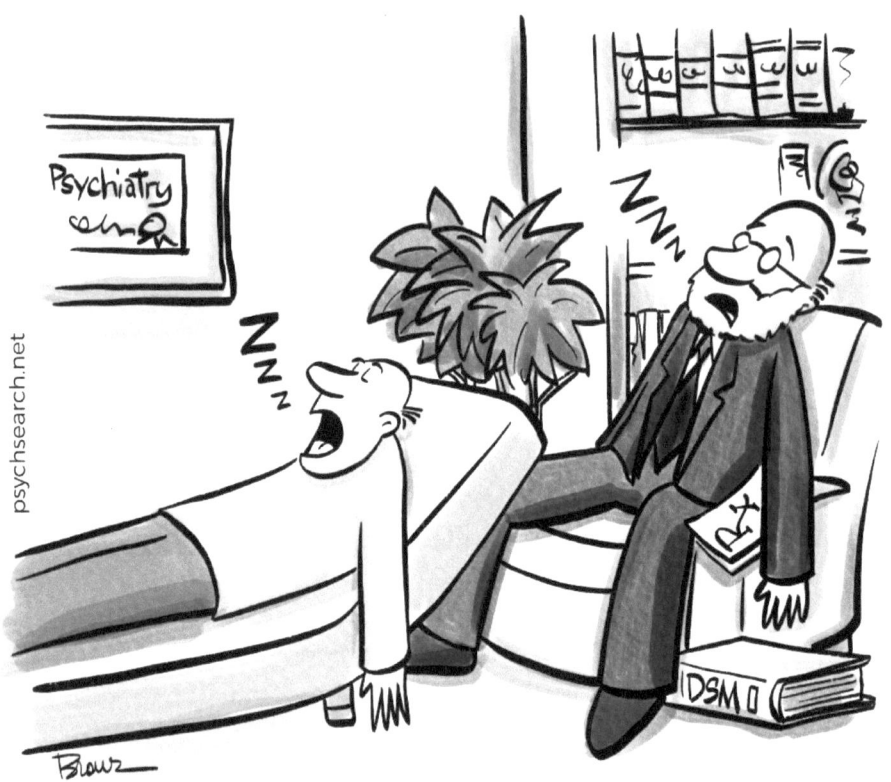

The "Shrink" Tank
by Verde
Psychsearch.net
DUNK-A-SHRINK
Verde
©2014 VERDE

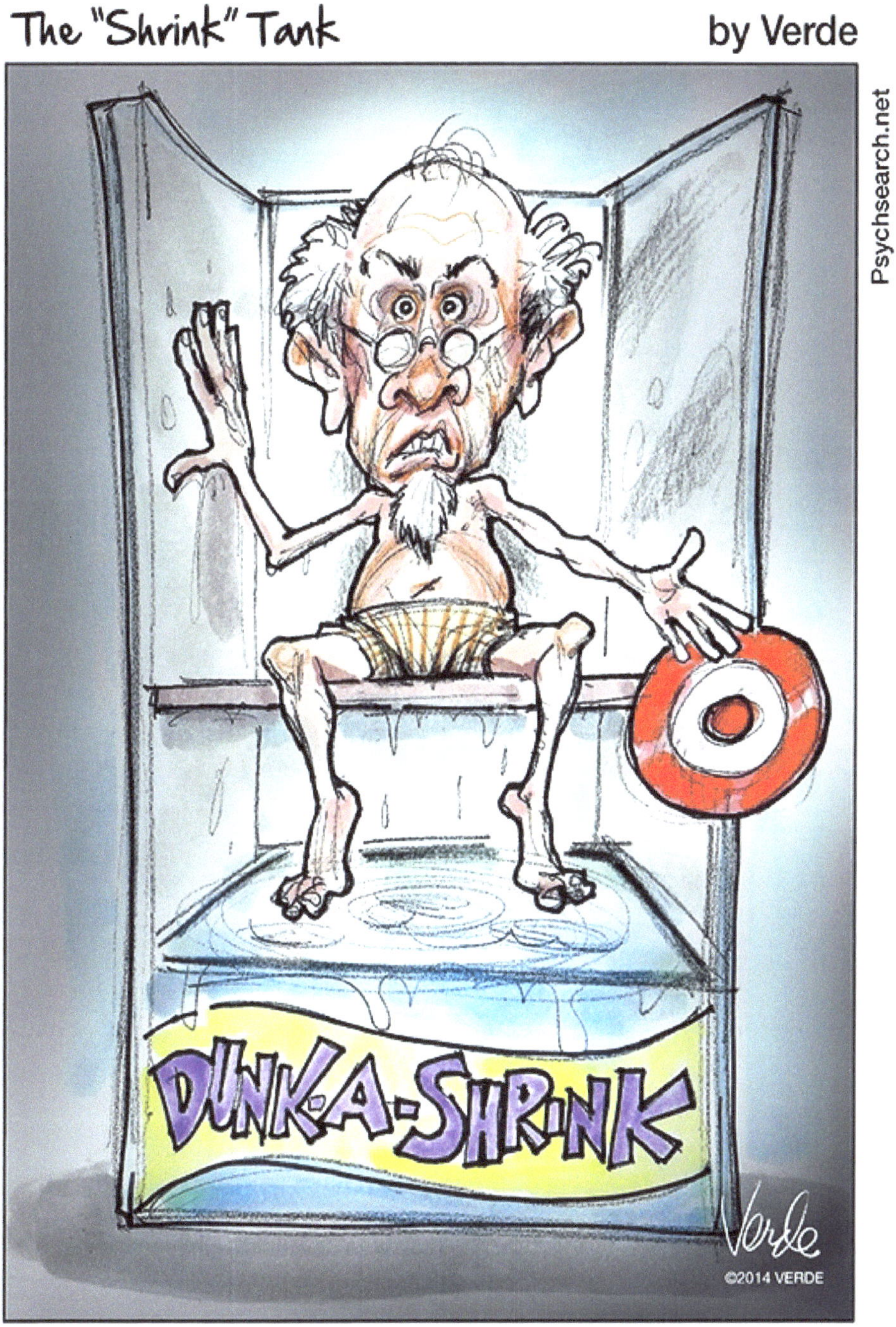

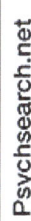

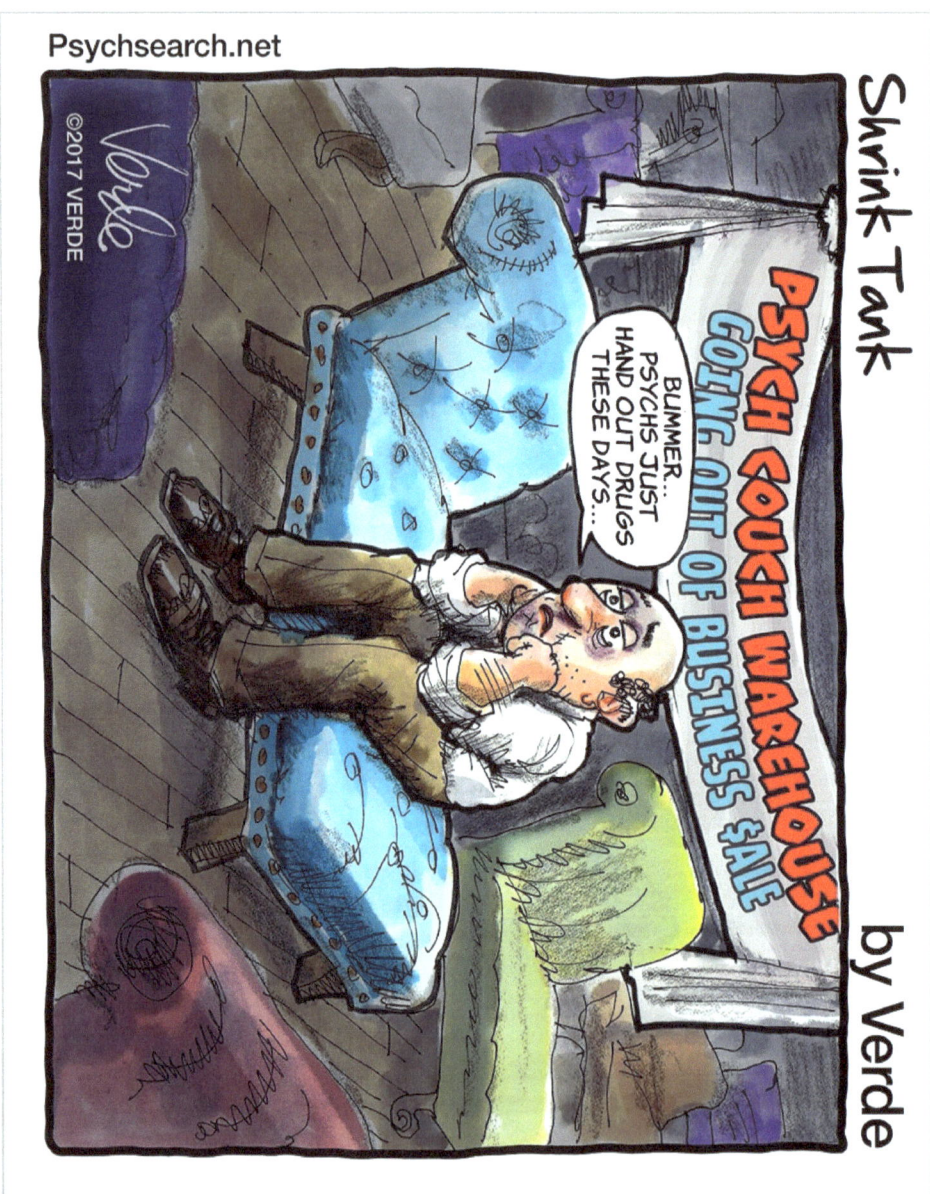

Psychs

by Kramer & Brown

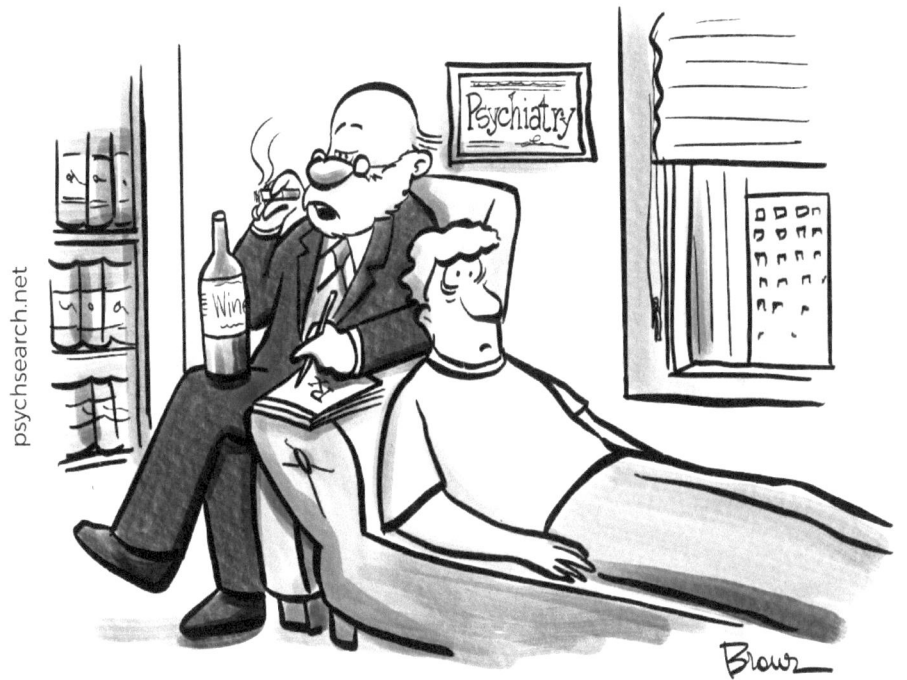

"PsychSearch just put my records on the net."

HOLIDAYS

The "Shrink" Tank

by Verde

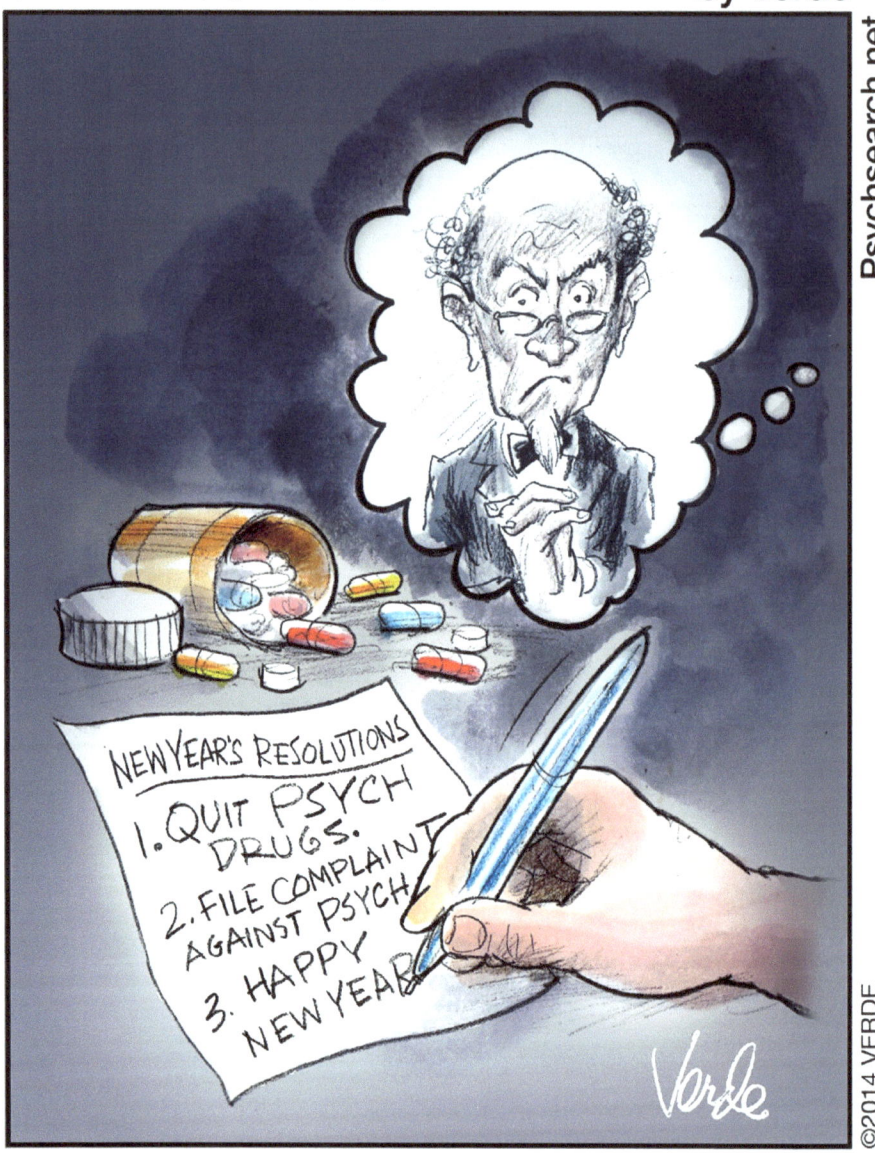

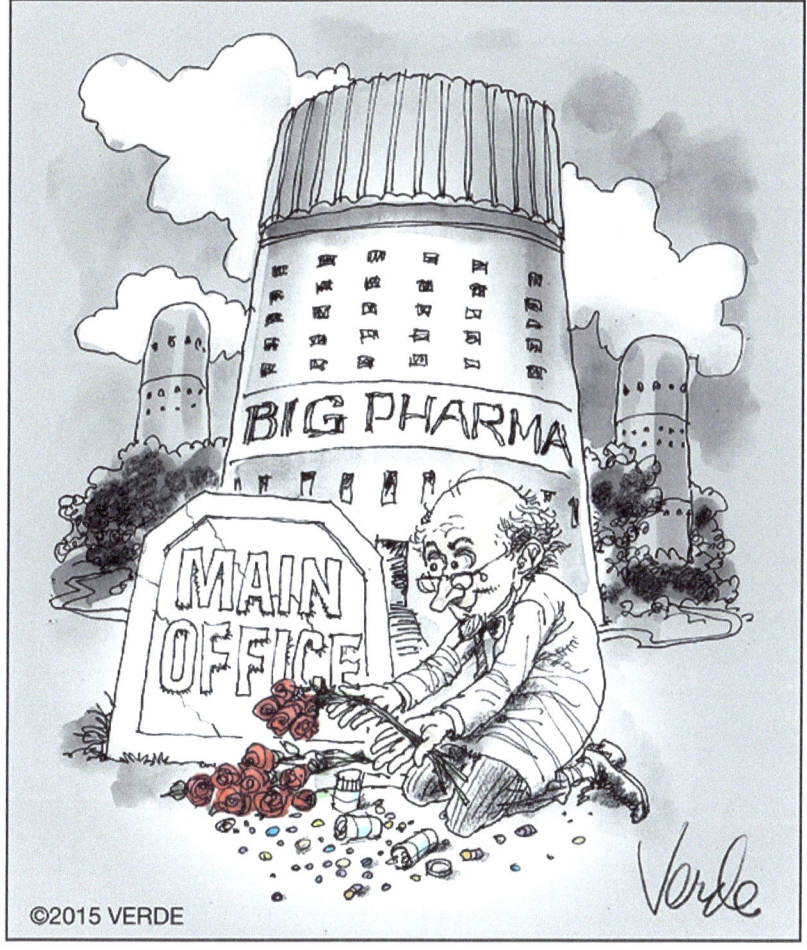

Psychiatrist's Valentine's Day

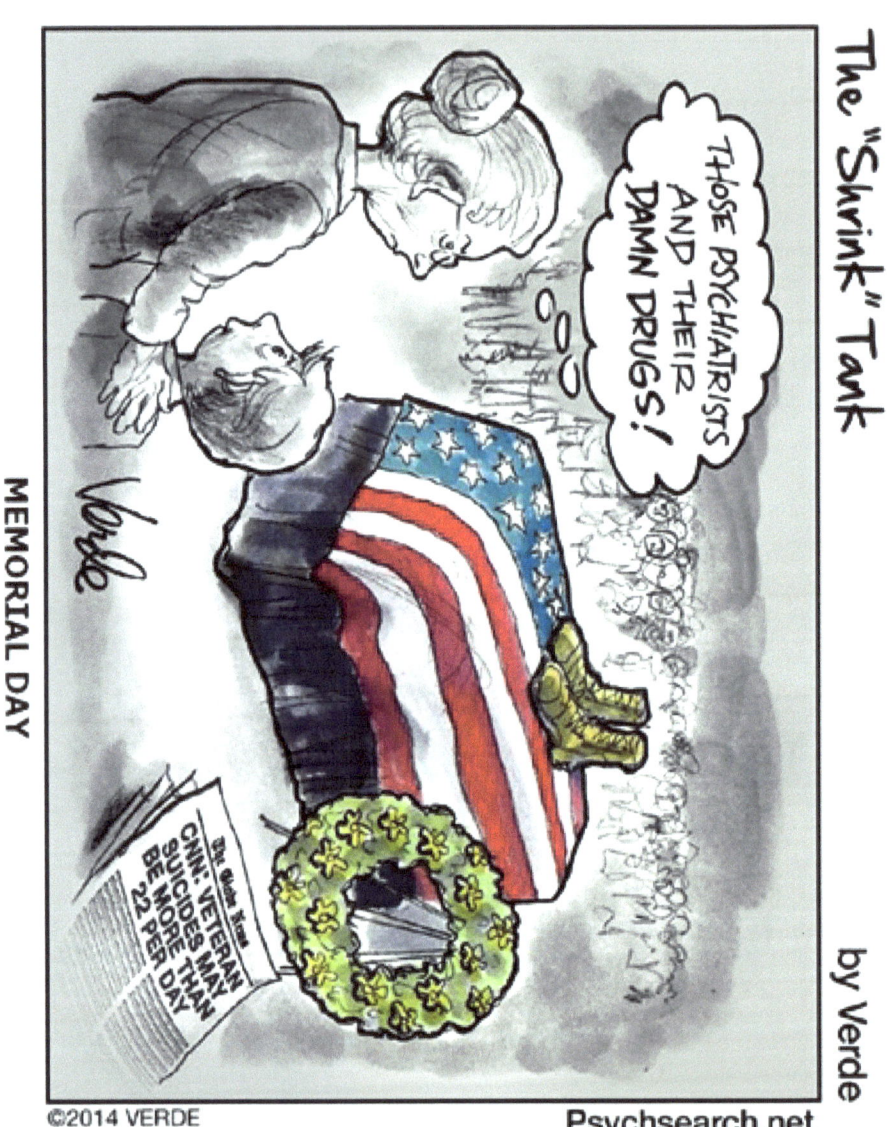

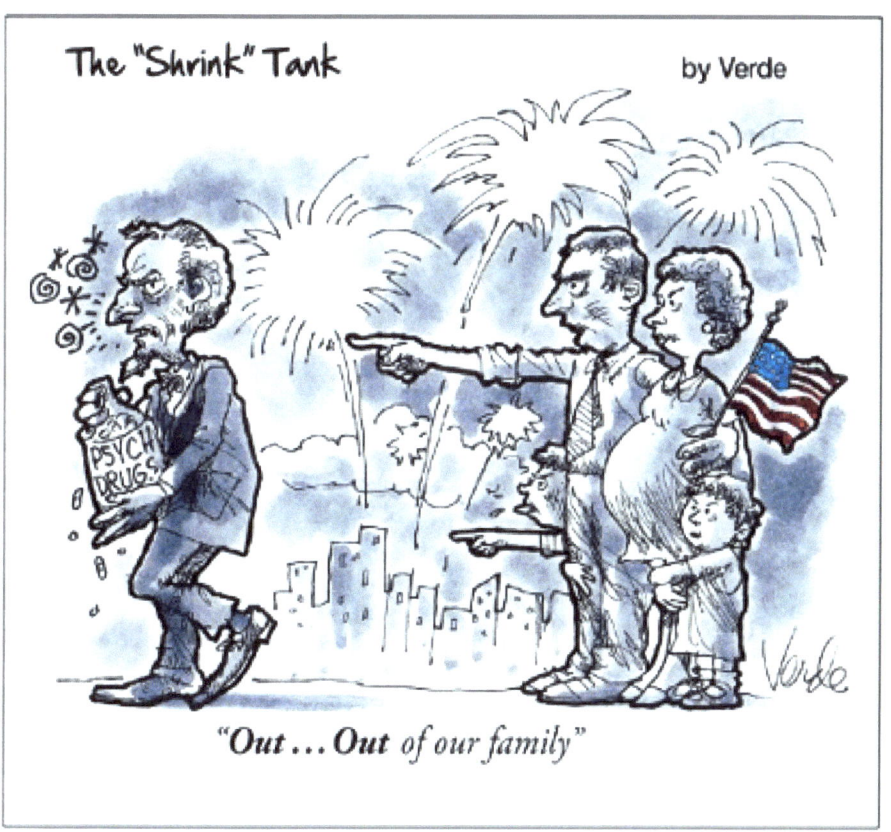

Psychsearch.net

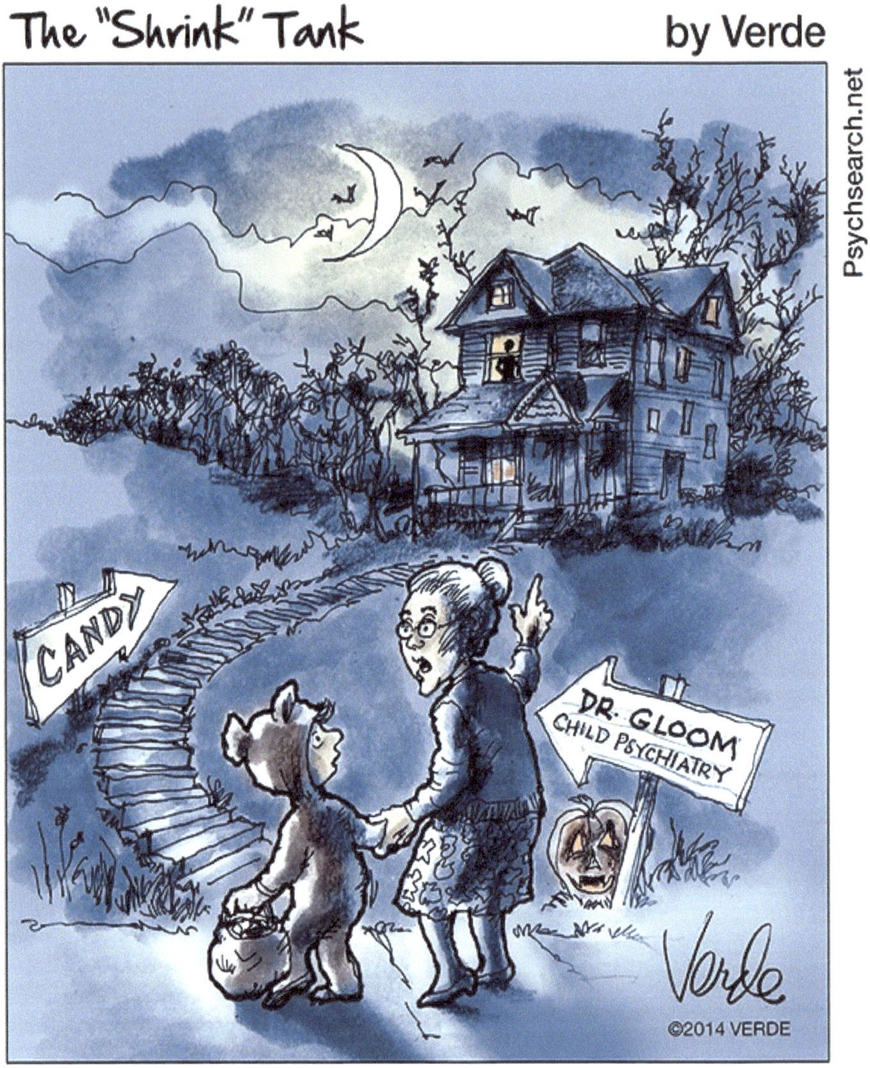

The "Shrink" Tank
by Verde
Psychsearch.net
CANDY
DR. GLOOM
CHILD PSYCHIATRY
Verde
©2014 VERDE

"No, honey! Psychiatrists only hand out drugs!"

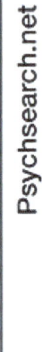

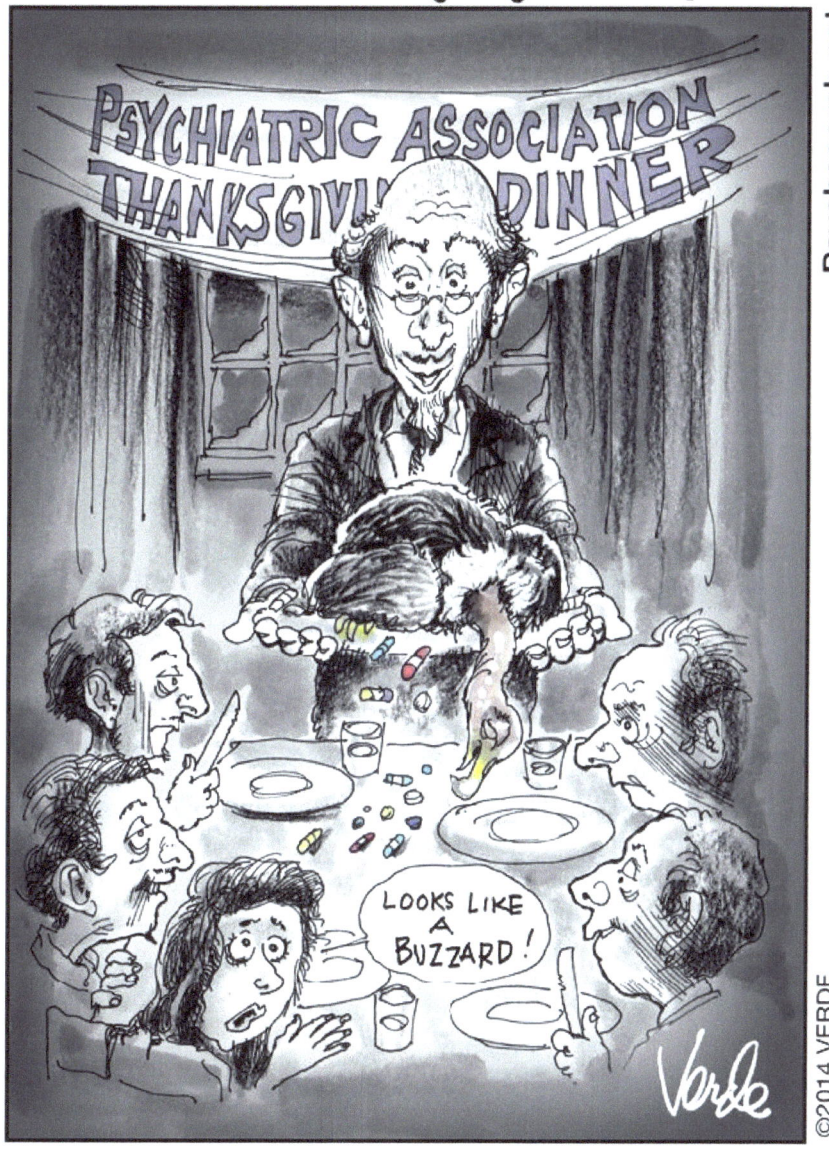

"Drug him. Commit him. Maybe even some electroconvulsive therapy."

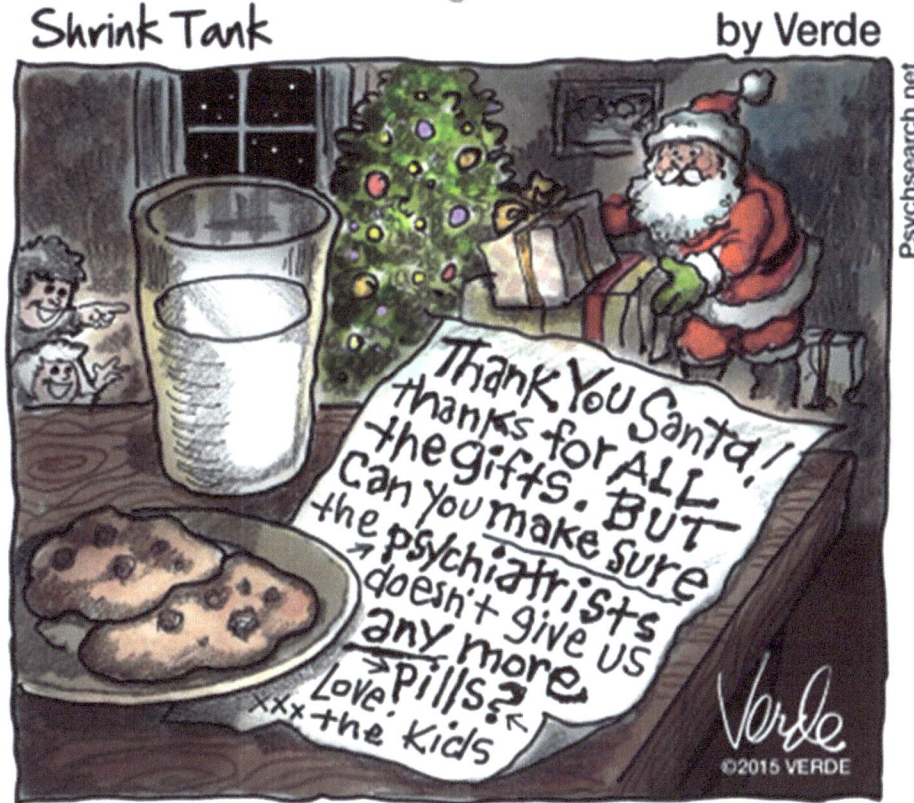

A Child's Wishlist for Santa

THE FUTURE

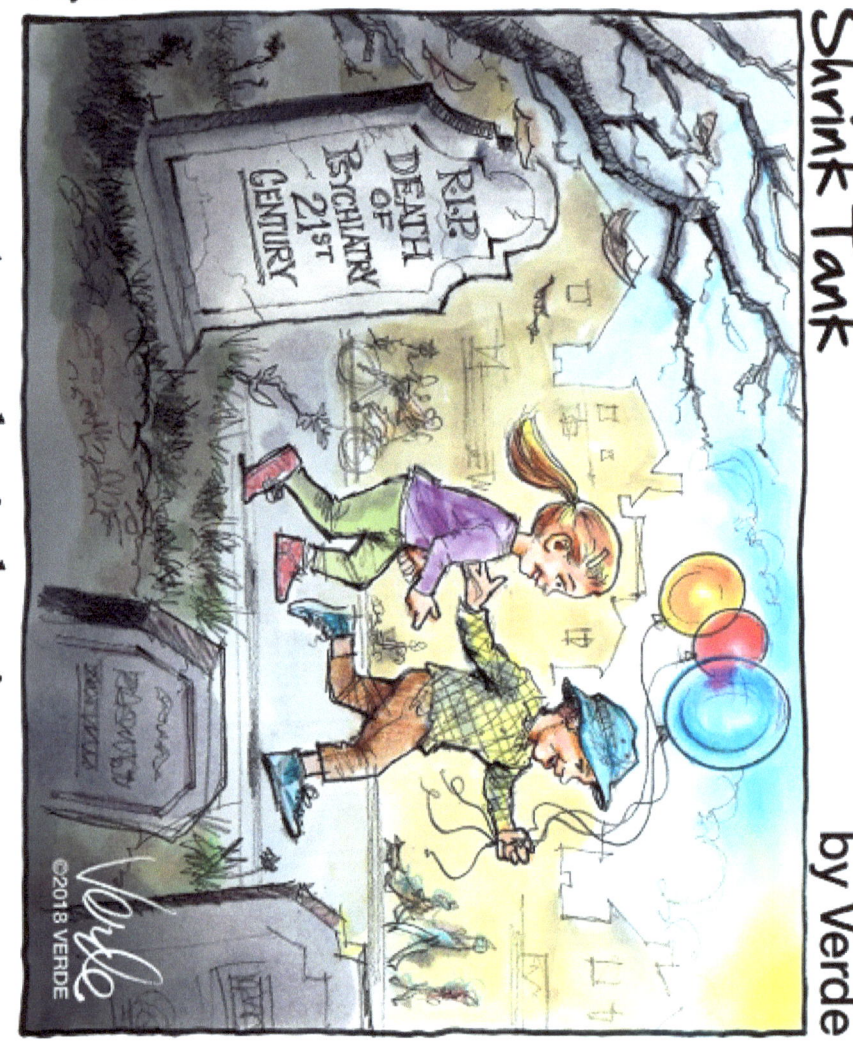

You can always write to me at records@psychsearch.net.

Thank you!

Kenneth Kramer

www.ingramcontent.com/pod-product-compliance
Lightning Source LLC
Chambersburg PA
CBHW041100180526
45172CB00001B/36